Neurological Assessment
During the First Year of Life

Neurological
Assessment
During the First Year of Life

CLAUDINE AMIEL-TISON, M.D.
Associate Professor of Pediatrics
Baudelocque Maternity Hospital, Paris

ALBERT GRENIER, M.D.
Chief of Service, Department of Pediatrics
Bayonne City Hospital, France

Translated by
ROBERTA GOLDBERG, M.D.

New York   Oxford
OXFORD UNIVERSITY PRESS
1986

Oxford University Press

Oxford   New York   Toronto
Delhi   Bombay   Calcutta   Madras   Karachi
Petaling Jaya   Singapore   Hong Kong   Tokyo
Nairobi   Dar es Salaam   Cape Town
Melbourne   Auckland

and associated companies in
Beirut   Berlin   Ibadan   Nicosia

Translated from *La Surveillance neurologique au cours de la première année*
de la vie by Claudine Amiel-Tison, M.D., and Albert Grenier, M.D. Copyright
© Masson, Editeur, Paris, 1984.

Copyright © 1986 by Claudine Amiel-Tison, M.D., and Albert Grenier, M.D.

Published by Oxford University Press, Inc.
200 Madison Avenue, New York, New York, 10016

Oxford is a registered trademark of Oxford University Press.

Library of Congress Cataloging-in-Publication Data
Amiel-Tison, Claudine.
Neurological assessment during the first year of life.
Translation of: La surveillance neurologique au cours
de la première année de la vie.
Includes bibliographies and index.
1. Nervous system—Diseases—Diagnosis.
2. Infants (Newborn)—Diseases—Diagnosis.
3. Infants (Premature)—Diseases—Diagnosis.
4. Neurologic examination.
I. Grenier, Albert.   II. Title.   [DNLM: 1. Infant, Newborn.
2. Infant, Premature.   3. Neurologic Examination—
in infancy & childhood.   4. Nervous System Diseases—diagnosis.
5. Nervous System Diseases—in infancy & childhood.   WS 340 A516s]
RJ290.5.A4513   1986   618.92'80475   85-25957
ISBN 0-19-504029-5

9 8 7 6 5 4 3 2 1
Printed in the United States of America
on acid-free paper

FOREWORD

The contributions of Dr. Amiel-Tison over the past two decades have crystallized the concept of a predictable sequence of neurological development in early infancy. Her data constitute so important a foundation in the neurology of the postnatal period that they complete the chapter of medical history that began with perinatal studies by her Parisian predecessors André Thomas and Saint-Anne Dargassies. Dr. Amiel-Tison has been honored by the most meaningful of compliments that can be offered to a scientific investigator: her work repeatedly has been confirmed and restated by some of the most celebrated neurologists in England, the United States, and other countries. Albert Grenier has equally earned the respect of his colleagues in infant physiotherapy and rehabilitation throughout the world by his many original contributions over the years to this discipline.

This concise monograph summarizes and integrates the meticulous observations of these two dedicated physicians, formulating their data into thoughtful generalizations, at times evoking imaginative interpretations. Trends and patterns in neurological development are thus identified. Not only is there a caudocephalic gradient of acquisition of muscle tone and motor functions in the premature infant and neonate, but the gradient then reverses during the first year, becoming a cephalocaudal progression of further motor control, with upper extremity skills accelerating faster than those of the lower limbs. The progressive equalization of flexor and extensor tone in axial muscles during the final three months of gestation, as described by Saint-Anne Dargassies, are emphasized in the light of subsequent acquisition of head control, sitting, standing, and other clinical expressions of axial muscle control.

Transitory abnormalities in motor function during the first year are used as a basis for risk indicators of later minor motor neurological impairment, with implications not only in delayed fine motor skills but also in intellectual function and behavior during the school years. Thus, the continuity between perinatal insult and minimal handicaps in childhood is bridged. Neuromotor and cognitive abilities and "communication" by the infant provide a sound basis for predicting, within limits, the projected cerebral functions of later childhood. Attention to and imitation of facial gestures by the young infant are cited as examples of neonatal awareness of the environment. These "evoked states of communication" and "liberated motricity" of Dr. Grenier are valuable signs both for reassuring anxious parents of high-risk infants and for identifying those children who might be suitable candidates for preschool intervention programs. Social development of the infant in subsequent months is a direct extension of these early environmental interactions, dependent upon and closely intertwined with sensory and motor development.

The original French-language edition is so beautifully written that it evoked anxiety to contemplate it in translation, but the excellent English version has lost none of the clear and systematic development of themes. The carefully selected photographs, line drawings, and tables serve to further illuminate the practical applications of the descriptive and theoretical material presented by illustrating the various postures, reflexes, and maneuvers of physical examination. The Appendix provides a systematic scheme for assessing the features of physical examination described.

I am honored to be invited by these distinguished authors to introduce their illuminating conclusions, derived from years of painstaking observations, notes, and analyses.

Harvey B. Sarnat
Calgary, Canada

PREFACE

What is new in neonatal neurology that justifies all the attention it is getting? More than can be imagined has occurred in this discipline that for a long time had been reduced to the unfortunate task of keeping track of the sequelae of perinatal difficulties.

In the first place, the extension of perinatal care to the group of newborns weighing <1000 g is a recent phenomenon that has made it even more important to have feedback on the outcome for low birth weight (LBW) newborns. The long-term results should permit obstetricians to improve their indications for termination of a pregnancy at risk. The epidemiologists should be better able to evaluate the parallel trends of mortality and morbidity: are these trends continuing as in the past, or is mortality decreasing while morbidity is increasing in the very low birth weight (VLBW) infant? The economists will have the data to make cost–benefit studies. The recent results for the group from 800 to 1000 g are surprising, because they show that morbidity is comparable to the heavier group of 1000 to 1500 g in incidence and nature, while neonatal mortality in the lower birth weight group is much higher.

In the second place, transfontanellar echography has become part of daily life in intensive care during the past few years. The oldest children who had the benefit of this evaluation as a newborn are now approaching school age; echoclinical correlation is therefore well advanced. This ability to evaluate the infant without transfer, fatigue or additional risk, to evaluate intracranial hemmorhage with precision, to see the evolution from the first weeks to the first months of life, has given new life to the clinicomorphological approach. The neurological evaluation could not very well lag behind the morphological investigation; it had to advance as well and become more precise. Clinical evaluation is still more reliable than currently available imaging in detecting minor neurological deficits.

In the third place, recent research on the extraordinary neurosensorial competence of the newborn allows clinicians to be more demanding in defining normality at this age and therefore more precise in defining the group at risk. In effect, early affirmation of normalcy has become possible in more and more newborns, and therefore this decreases the number of infants considered to be at risk.

In 1950 Gesell described the newborn: "The poor babe like a seaman wrecked, thrown from the waves, lies naked o'er the ground."

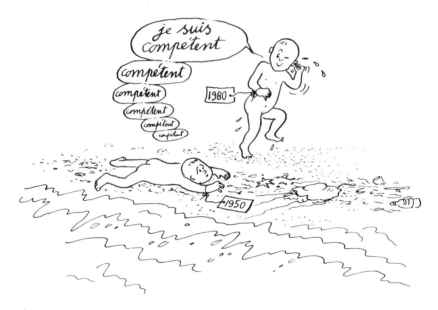

More than 30 years later, still naked but competent, the newborn of the 1980s can demonstrate amazing abilities and can interact with the family and medical team.

One of the primary effects of this progress in the evaluation of the newborn has been the early prevention of psychological disorders in the family of the infant "at risk." This represents a complete change of attitude by the medical team: with the improvement in long-term outcome and more refined clinical and imaging methods, the medical team is now ready to ask each newborn to demonstrate his or her normal neuromotor function as early as possible. When the responses are not perfect, evaluations will continue in the presence of the parents, who follow the progressive appearance of motor and behavioral acquisitions with the medical team. And when the newborn becomes interested in the examination, when there is appropriate sensorial stimulation the result can be the infant's active participation, which can even allow the examiner to anticipate motor normalization. Since intense interaction by the infant is an essential prerequisite to the infant's performance, there is a strong temptation to infer that cognitive function will be normal as well.

The value of this early demonstration of intact abilities in a convalescing newborn greatly surpasses the examiner's immediate satisfaction in eliciting these responses. For the parents this demonstration is worth a thousand words. It is frequently only after such a demonstration that the parents dare to truly interact with their newborn. In the rare cases where normalcy cannot be demonstrated and instead after the first months of doubt, there are evident sequelae, the interaction that has already been established will be a major asset for the handicapped child. Whether there is handicap or not, it must be appreciated that this interaction, this positive and rich give-and-take between two individuals, is not always present in all families. It is not major problems that pose the only danger to this interaction; often when there are only minor difficulties it is most important to reinforce this relationship over the years.

The interest in noting *transient motor anomalies* is to try to identify these cases as early as possible, so as to assure that the problems of adaptation through school age are understood and accepted. When fine motor activity and/or intellectual functions are affected, even at a minor level, the problems will begin to be evident at school age. The children and their families go through a very painful period of adjustment. They must be well informed that these difficulties may represent an ongoing burden for everyone involved; the parent–child interaction must be constantly reinforced. In this very hazy area of "minimal brain dysfunction" (MBD), it is essential to avoid the frequently passionate opposition between the two schools of thought, organic and psychogenic; less traditional and more inventive methods of assistance must be sought. After an unsuccessful first year at school we often see parents return to their neonatologist with a child of 7 or 8 years; they are seeking help, guidance, and hope from their first doctor with the feeling that these problems are likely the result of perinatal events. It is a shame that what they are seeking was not given to them preventively, with the same continuous support that is given to a more seriously handicapped child and family.

An important aspect of the role of the neonatologist is to understand the limits of the role. When severe handicap becomes overtly evident to both the neonatologist and the family, the situation has reached the point that it is both necessary and acceptable to everyone involved for the neonatologist to "pass the baton" to specialists for the overall management of the child's care.

The neurological examination of the newborn and infant has not always been as well accepted as it is today. The progress of neonatology and the rapid development of early intervention have contributed to the acceleration of this phenomenon. When greater numbers of newborns began to survive intensive care, the anxiety was such that motor sequelae were assumed to be present until proven otherwise. With the passing of time, this attitude has been rapidly modified. It has become routine when examining a former 1-kg premature who has reached the age of term, after a very difficult course of respiratory distress, multiple pneumothoraxes, intraventricular hemorrhage, ligature of a ductus, and bronchopulmonary dysplasia to find normal neurological criteria for the age: contact, visual pursuit, and normal motor function. This initial evaluation, which is done on discharge from the intensive care unit, does not allow for the affirmation of subsequent normalcy. The infant will be regularly followed during the first year by classical methods of neuromotor and psychomotor evaluation.

Some facts can be summarized as follows:

1. Cerebral motor handicap is rare. This diagnosis can be made from around 3 to 4 months of age in its severe form. However, it is more often necessary to use more specific tests to recognize and affirm such a handicap before undertaking a program of rehabilitation.

2. By contrast, transient neuromotor anomalies are frequent during the first year. It is likely that they are minor lesions that have a maximum motor expression between 6 and 8 months corrected age and then disappear with ongoing maturation of the central nervous system (CNS). They would have no prognostic value if a close correlation were not being established between these transient motor anomalies and difficulties in adaptation to school. It is most likely that the clinical expression of moderate cellular lesions of various topographical locations changes with growth: first motor anomalies, then language problems, behavioral problems, and finally fine motor and intellectual deficits at school age. The observation of this progression reinforces the importance of continued surveillance of children who have had transient neuromotor anomalies in their first year.

3. When neuromotor anomalies are found during the first year, it is

still extremely difficult to *differentiate* those that will be transient from those that will result in sequelae; the complementary neuromotor examination (CNME) was designed to provide an early separation of the two groups: those who will rapidly normalize and those who will likely have permanent symptomatology of various expression.

The logical approach therefore becomes as follows: it is not useful to continue to examine newborns at risk as if they were carriers of the germ for a severe motor handicap. It would be most helpful to decrease the number of cases of infants suspected of having a cerebral motor handicap.

Practically speaking, the following sequence of actions is necessary:

- Affirm normal motor function from the first weeks of life by studying this motor action.
- Detect various anomalies that may be transient during the regular monthly exams throughout the first year.
- In the absence of such anomalies, relax the follow-up at the end of 1 year.
- By contrast, when anomalies are found continue surveillance even after secondary normalization.
- Concentrate all the various possible medical and educational resources on these children for whom subsequent risk of minor handicap is established.

The methods of evaluation we have proposed represent only some *components* of a complete neurological evaluation; we have chosen those methods that correspond to our current research. Each maneuver suggested is fully described and the different responses analyzed. The aspects of interpretation are then discussed. Claudine Amiel-Tison uses a grid to summarize the most common transient anomalies observed during the first year of life in order to establish a solid base for long-term prognosis. Albert Grenier has proposed a complementary neuromotor examination to be done from the first weeks of life when nothing is certain, nothing definite—an examination that in spite of any unfavorable clinical appearances would allow for the affirmation of the complete preservation of neuromotor potential, on which basis he eliminates the possibility of major cerebral motor handicap and predicts the ability to walk. The contribution of these methods toward early prognosis of cognitive function remains to be shown.

Our thanks to Annette Tison, who has graciously put her talent at our disposition. Her illustrations reproduce the movements of babies with such purity of style that we are often led to reevaluate our descriptions, which seem imprecise.

Our gratitude to the personnel at the Centre Hospitalier de Bayonne and the Centre de Rééducation Motrice pour Enfants Infirmes Moteurs Cérébraux "Aintzina," and especially to Anne-Marie Dezoteux, physio-therapist, who is always at the side of our convalescing newborns and their parents.

We express our special gratitude to Bernadette Valpreda, our secretary, who never waivered in making endless corrections on this manuscript: her sense of the English language and her passion for perfection only partially explain her dedication.

Roberta Goldberg came to France for a visit and, like Ulysses, stayed for years. She learned French and newborn neurology. We realize how lucky we have been to have had the benefit of her expertise in this translation; we enjoyed working with her and hope that she will return to France for another "visit."

Finally, we want to thank Daniel Osherson, professor at the Massachusetts Institute of Technology. He gave us confidence that our French version merited translation, thereby providing us with the necessary encouragement to persist.

Paris   C. A-T.
May 1986   A.G.

CONTENTS

Neurological Assessment
During the First Year of Life

1

DEVELOPMENTAL NEUROLOGY: New Demands

Developmental neurology is a continuously growing discipline. Having taken its place between classical pediatric neurology and child psychology, it has become an important area of psychological research. The study of neurological development has at the same time diversified, expanded, and become more precise. It must now be able to respond to multiple demands: those of the obstetrician, the neuropsychiatrist, and, most important, those of the parents. Parents now play an active role in postnatal follow-up care, as they do during the hospitalization of their newborn. Everything possible must be done to ease their anxiety during their child's first months of life.

The Obstetrician's Point of View

More than ever, obstetricians need short-term feedback on the results of the neurological evaluation of the infants they deliver, as there are now many more very low birth weight (VLBW) infants being delivered. In the continuing decision-making process, outcome is an essential factor. The decision when to deliver a fetus at risk may result in neonatal death, the survival of an infant with a major or minor handicap, or ideally a healthy infant. Therefore, obstetricians must have an understanding of the results for different etiological factors. Two examples of how obstetricians benefit from knowing the outcome are chronic fetal distress and malignant illness of the pregnant woman.

The subject of *chronic fetal distress* is extremely complex due to the diversity of causes for the distress: chronic maternal disease, maternal disease secondary to the pregnancy, or a disorder of unknown etiology. The examples of essential hypertension or preclampsia are indicative

3

of the problems faced by obstetricians, who must seek the best solution taking into account the sometimes conflicting interests of the pregnant woman and the fetus. After becoming aware of the maternal signs and symptoms, the obstetrician evaluates the well-being of the fetus by fetal heart monitoring and evaluates its growth by clinical and ultrasound measurements. These parameters are essential parts of the decision as to when the benefit of intrauterine growth development is outweighed by the risk of compromised vascular supply (best judged by fetal heart monitoring) [1,2]. Deciding to wait risks not only fetal death but the survival of an infant with cerebral sequelae. The obstetrician must calculate the risk between prenatal complications *in utero* and postnatal complications secondary to prematurity, for example respiratory distress syndrome (RDS) or intraventricular hemorrhage. He or she will consult the recent literature [3] and will be greatly aided by feedback from the institution in trying to determine the risk of mortality or sequelae. For VLBW infants, obstetrics has gone beyond the realm of the unknown. Obstetricians now have the uneasy and disquieting ability to make a rational choice based on the new methods of antenatal exploration and postnatal care. It is hoped that in the future their investigations can go even further: in what way is the slowing of craniocerebral growth (measured by ultrasound) linked to unfavorable cerebral prognosis [4,5]?

Another example illustrates the problem from a different aspect, that of *the pregnant woman with a malignancy*. When the diagnosis is made after the fifth month of pregnancy, in what way can the interests of all best be served: of the pregnant woman who needs immediate treatment, and of the fetus who can support life but is at great risk due to its extreme immaturity? Actually between 26 and 30 weeks, the curve of mortality is a function of gestational age (GA); for a mean birth weight it is almost vertical (Fig. 1-1), so that one additional week can drastically change the prognosis for the fetus. However, by comparison much less is gained by waiting until between 30 and 34 weeks. It is the goal of graphs such as the one reproduced in Figure 1-1 to give the obstetrician a rational basis for decision making [6].

The curves of neonatal mortality must be associated with curves of neurological morbidity. Without these curves the alternative is to indicate the trends observed in long-term analysis of the recent literature. For example, in the study of Knobloch *et al.* [7] at the Perinatal Center in Albany, New York, the analysis of results for a period of nearly 30 years showed that improvements in perinatal and neonatal care have resulted in the same outcome at present for newborns be-

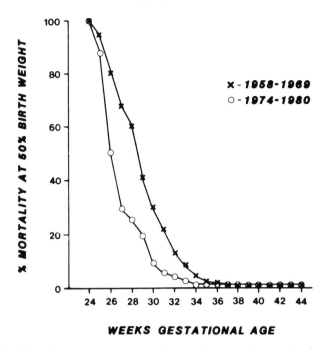

Fig. 1-1 Plot of neonatal mortality risk as a function of gestational age for a birth weight at the 50th percentile. Comparison of data from the period 1958–1969 and from the period 1974–1980.
(From Koops B. L., Morgan L. J. and Battaglia F. C. *J. Pediatr.*, *101*, 969–977, 1982, with permission.)

tween 750 and 1000 g birth weight that were obtained in 1952 for newborns of birth weight between 1000 and 1500 g. In 1952, the mortality compared to previous years decreased significantly in the group of newborns between 1000 and 1500 g who received excellent care but no assisted ventilation, but only half the survivors were normal. It should be noted that morbidity in this group decreased with the introduction of assisted ventilation.

Because of the importance of this information to their daily decision making, obstetricians can be given a prognosis based on a very rough summary of current data, noting the existence of significant national and regional variation. that is, for the group of newborns of birth weight between 800 and 1500 g, 10–15% of the survivors risk major cerebral sequelae. For birth weight <800 g the cerebral prognosis for the survivors is moderate to poor despite excellent quality intensive care [8,9].

The great interest in the group of infants of birth weight <1500 g, as in the two examples above, should not overshadow the fact that all newborns, no matter what their birth weight, can develop problems. There is very low risk in the birth of a eutrophic infant at term only in the well-staffed, well-equipped centers where emergencies can be swiftly handled and fetal monitoring is used for *all deliveries.* It is only with an attitude of permanent attentiveness to "normal" low-risk pregnancies that birth accidents can be eliminated. However, this is not the case at present, and it will not likely ever be universal; as a result, there are a significant number of infants with major handicaps as a result of intrapartum asphyxia. Eliminating this sequelae is the daily battle of obstetrics—a battle that is perhaps less glamorous than saving a tiny preterm infant, yet one that is essential for optimal outcome in the entire newborn population.

The Parent's Point of View

The high-risk pregnancy is a very difficult period for the future parents, who in effect live with the obstetrician during this difficult period of choices leading up to the delivery of their infant. The pregnant woman often accepts a long prenatal hospitalization and a caesarian section with only a vague understanding of the respective risks to her fetus of mortality and survival with sequelae. It is implicit for these parents that everything be done to save their infant. The parents are often aware of the statistics, but they continue to have determination and tremendous hope that their infant will fall on the right side of the data. They do not want to hear pessimistic if realistic forecasts: it is only their great hope that allows them to create a bond with their infant during the long separation. Our experience is that this hope is well founded; the prediction of sequelae is often excessive within the first year of life, as is described below. Also, because there is little that can be done for a significantly damaged brain, little is to be gained by knowing that information early.

It is difficult to measure the effect of perinatal events on the mother–infant relationship in a rigorous fashion. It has, however, been attempted [10,11,12,13]. The study of factors that shape the mother's opinion of her baby's development show that birth weight, hospitalizations in the first year, significant disorder, and congenital malformations reinforce the image of a sickly and vulnerable child. This way of looking at her child can have a long-term effect on the mother–child interaction and can thus unfavorably influence the subsequent development of the child.

The Neonatologist's Point of View

For the tiny premature newborn, the acute period of the first few weeks is followed by a period of convalescence during which further difficulties frequently occur: vasomotor instability, respiratory function affected by complications secondary to pulmonary immaturity and assisted ventilation, feeding problems, and metabolic adjustments.

With the start of the period of convalescence, a short neurological examination becomes possible. That is, several maneuvers used to evaluate passive and active tone become feasible and will complement the basic observations of the behavior and spontaneous activity of the infant. Tolerance for these maneuvers is often poor because of easy fatigability and cardiorespiratory instability. Signs of transient intracranial hypertension (ICH) are not rare as a result of an increase in extracellular fluid secondary to inadequate elimination of sodium in cases of high oral intake [14,15]. Interpreted outside the context of an excessive weight gain, these signs of ICH are unnecessarily alarming; however, it is useful to pick up these signs to initiate the appropriate action to reverse them. It would similarly be important to note insufficient hydration with significant overriding of sutures in an infant who has inadequate head circumference growth from purely nutritional origin. It is imperative that any neurological evaluation, to be satisfactory, take into account the ongoing medical context.

Orthopedic evaluation of the infant is similarly dependent on the disorder(s) the infant has experienced during the acute period. After weeks of inadequate nutrition and fixation on a hard flat surface, the articulations are painful and the posture abnormal. The consequences of these conditions worsen if they are not corrected early. The motor apparatus must be returned to proper function by manipulation and stimulation. It is useless to try to draw conclusions on long-term prognosis based on early evaluations. These considerations lead to the following conclusions.

1. *The neonatologist can make a valid neurological evaluation of a convalescing newborn but must take into account the situation of the infant as a whole.* This is also true for the neurologist who is part of the neonatal team; the neurologist who is not familiar with neonatology and comes from another environment will not be able to make such an evaluation. The examiner must take into account respiratory and metabolic contingencies, must observe the infant over a period of time, and must repeat the evaluation frequently at favorable moments in the

day. The period of convalescence continues from the first weeks of growth until the first months at home. During this time there is great variability of signs. By definition a period of convalescence is not one of definite limits; the existence and/or severity of handicaps cannot be evaluated until the period of stabilization has been attained [16].

2. *It is only significant to note positive actions during the period of convalescence.* Experience has long shown that normal neuromotor function as evaluated near 40 weeks corrected age is essentially a guarantee of subsequent normalcy and can be very reassuring for the prognosis of the infant [17]. That is to say, an infant at 40 weeks corrected age who has attained normal head circumference, has normal sutures [18], good visual perception and good attentiveness [19], and normal motor performance has every reason to grow and develop normally. However, the inverse is not true. Many initial neurological anomalies do not have predictive value [20], aside from serious dysfunction like hydrocephalus, significant opisthotonos, inadequate head circumference growth, absence of visual perception, and absence of contact; many moderate anomalies of reflexes and tone are not correlated with future dysfunction. This is also the experience described by Hunt [21].

The data available from the neurological examination of newborns up to 40 weeks corrected age was restudied and compared with ultrasound data by Stewart *et al.* [22,23]. They found that with a normal ultrasound the neurological examination at 40 weeks is helpful to confirm the identification of normal infants, but when the ultrasound findings are abnormal the clinical examination will not help predict outcome. The best prediction of an unfavorable future comes from ultrasound evidence of an increase in the size of the lateral ventricles (cerebral atrophy).

3. *Improvement of the clinical neurological evaluation must be geared toward early confirmation of normalcy and not toward signs that may predict sequelae.* It is through the demonstration of a series of active motor events that neuromotor integrity can be affirmed. This is particularly true for infants who have anomalies on the classical examination. In order to identify as early as possible in the period of convalescence the infants who will develop normally, the clinical investigation must go into as much detail as possible. In addition to this clinical evaluation, ultrasound and electroencephalographic (EEG) monitoring are used when indicated.

4. *This type of careful monitoring should extend to all newborns.* The efforts of saving VLBW newborns occupy much of the energy of intensive care centers. It must be noted, however, that for "normal"

newborns labor room observation and the evaluation during the first days of life are essential for the prevention of cerebral sequelae in the population as a whole. In the same way early detection of infection has decreased neonatal meningitis, monitoring of jaundice has almost eliminated the neurosensorial effects of hyperbilirubinemia, and the detection of apnea has diminished cerebral ischemic damage.

The neurological examination is so valuable for the eutrophic full-term newborn that when the findings are normal in the first days of life the examiner can confirm that the circumstances of birth, even those less than optimal, have had no effect on future cerebral function. The Apgar score, for example, cannot then always be held responsible for subsequent functional deficits. Inversely, the conditions of birth may have been totally normal and yet there are neurological signs present at birth; their origin most likely lies in antenatal stress or a cerebral malformation. The neurological evaluation is therefore essential, as is frequently discovered in cases under litigation. A neurosensorial score has been proposed to compare different obstetrical or anesthesia techniques [24]. It would give each chart a notation of *optimality* of the birth process.

The Physiotherapist's Point of View

The role of early intervention on the evaluation of a cerebral motor disability (CMD) is still a subject of debate. The various viewpoints were recently restated in "The Early Diagnosis of Cerebral Motor Disability: What for?" [16]. Certainly compensatory mechanisms exist for all cerebral functions and this "brain plasticity" is encouraged by stimulation and by appropriate environment [25]. However, when a motor tract is interrupted by white matter ischemic lesions that lack the possibility of healing, the inevitable result is mild or moderate motor dysfunction with no possibility of repair by physiotherapy even if started very early.

However, the fundamental role of the physiotherapist cannot be denied. In the first months, if the complementary neuromotor examination does not give satisfactory results even on repeated trials, the physiotherapist can work with the joints that are subject to abnormal muscle tension. This is particularly true for the hips and the shoulders, for which orthopedic correction is possible. He or she can work more intensively with the infants who after the age of 4 months retain anomalies of motor function and are at greater risk of developing a motor disability, but who may also experience improvements in motor function as maturation progresses. Using standard physiotherapeutic techniques, the therapist works to maintain optimal body function and optimal use of damaged structures. This early work with all "suspects" eliminates any gap in the treatment of children in whom a definite CMD is eventually confirmed.

The Neuropsychiatrist's Point of View

The neuropsychiatrist will often be asked to see a child at age 6–7 years for the first time because of difficulty adapting to school. The etiological analysis is retrospective and the link between adverse conditions and perinatal difficulty is often not possible to trace. The radiological tests are completely deceiving in these cases of moderate difficulty, since they do not have the anatomical correlation that can be seen with severe deficits [26]. The absence of findings should not be taken as proof of normalcy. Retrospective analysis of these subtle problems is often inconclusive. We give here three examples seen in medicine daily—the syndrome of minimal brain dysfunction (MBD), psychological disorders, and convulsions—and show their association with unfavorable perinatal conditions.

MINIMAL BRAIN DYSFUNCTION

There have been many stages in the development of an acceptable definition of and the notion of multiple etiologies for MBD.

The generally accepted definition of MBD makes an association between an attention deficit and a motor or a perceptual motor difficulty; the diagnosis is made on school-age children who have neither major intellectual nor major motor deficits. This fine motor difficulty persists for life.

Compensatory mechanisms exist, but the deficit will likely affect the school years severely and often influence the choice of career. A general review by Rutter [27] analyzes the two major theoretical definitions of MBD.

1. The idea of a continuum wherein MBD is only a mild variant of more severe disorders of motor and attention deficits resulting from some type of cerebral damage
2. The theory of a genetically determined and clinically homogeneous syndrome

Rutter has no doubt about the relationship between a subclinical cerebral lesion and MBD, with psychiatric difficulties often associated.

He does not see this as a homogeneous syndrome and doubts there is any genetic basis.

The respective involvement of different etiological factors in MBD is still the subject of heated debate. These arguments are complicated by the negative effect of unfavorable interactions between problem children and problem parents. A recent Swedish study [28] used a cohort of 3448 children 6 years of age, in public schools in Göteborg. Among them, with a clear predominance of boys, 340 had attention deficits (distractibility or behavior problems) combined with motor or perceptual motor deficits; 138 of these 340 children were subjects in a double-blind neuropsychiatric study. The Swedish Health Organization is such that information on the perinatal events, hereditary factors, and socioeconomic situation are available for all children studied as well as all the controls. Nonoptimal scores were calculated for each factor studied. The results were as follows:

- Genetic factors were more frequently present in the group with MBD (18 versus 4%).
- Unfavorable perinatal factors were more common in the group with MBD (31 versus 9%).
- Unfavorable psychological factors were often associated with the other factors, but social disadvantage itself was not a common etiological factor.

PSYCHOLOGICAL SEQUELAE

The problem of psychological sequelae is twofold: intellectual deficit and psychiatric disorder. A severe intellectual deficit or psychiatric disorder has long been accepted to be secondary to a cerebral lesion. This association is not as clear in a moderate disorder, however. A recent general review [29] analyzes the known facts and shows that the presence of a cerebral lesion is associated with a marked risk of deficit, either intellectual or psychiatric.

There is good correlation between the extent of the lesion and the degree of intellectual deficit. However, this "dose–effect" correlation has not been demonstrated in psychiatric disorders.

CONVULSIONS

It appears evident that a seizure disorder can be the complication of a cerebral lesion of perinatal origin. This is the case, for example, of an ischemic lesion in the sylvian region, which results in hemiplegia and a cortical epileptogenic focus. Similarly, an anoxic ischemic encephalopathy often results in microcephaly, seizures, quadriplegia, and mental retardation. The cause–effect relationship is also clear in very hypotrophic newborns who are very excitable during their first year and develop a seizure disorder in early childhood. In Fitzhardinge's study in 1972 of a group of hypotrophic infants born at term [30], 6% had a seizure disorder.

In many cases the link between perinatal events and future seizure disorder is only probable, and no abnormality will be seen on cerebral computerized tomographic (CT) scan.

The same difficulty of interpretation exists when an infant who is known to have had perinatal difficulty has a seizure with fever. The possibility of recurrence of seizures or the risk of a prolonged episode are unknown.

In conclusion, the concept of a lesional continuum with variable expression is very convincing and has a certain clinical logic; however, there are uncertainties in each specific case. Tests such as the CT scan offer little help. It is the clinical examination that is the most sensitive. It is important to *recognize all the intermediate links* between perinatal distress and the outcome at age 7, in order to take effective therapeutic action for the group of children at high risk. Seeking out the intermediate stages between birth and school age in the areas of psychomotor and language function will result in better and more specific assistance.

The Epidemiologist's Point of View

A recent study by a group of North American epidemiologists [31–33], analyzing the perinatal literature since the mid-1950s, rings a pessimistic note. For example, the authors conclude their study of mortality and neurological morbidity in the VLBW infant [32] by stating that "at the present time it is premature to conclude that changes in newborn care have either lowered or raised rates of impairment among surviving low birth weight infants."

By contrast, the authors of a portion of the literature that was included in this review [34] reach a conclusion that corresponds more closely to the changes neonatologists have noted since the mid-1960s: "Since 1960 the chances of healthy survival have trebled, whereas the handicap rate has remained stable and relatively low at 6–8% of VLBW births . . . No evidence was found that the falling mortality rate had been achieved at the expense of the salvage of an increasing proportion of children who were handicapped."

A more balanced conclusion on the outcome of neonatal care comes from a carefully executed analysis of the population of Göteborg, Sweden [35]. The results are reassuring both to the public and in centers of neonatal intensive care. Until the beginning of the 1970s, in this area, perinatal mortality diminished and cerebral motor disabilities decreased, which led to a net increase in normal infants. From 1971 to 1975 the improvement in mortality figures continued (2100 more survivors), but the "cost" has been an increase in moderate cerebral motor disabilities (55 additional cases) without impaired intellectual function. "With the modern, very active neonatal care in Sweden the incidence of cerebral palsy has not decreased since the 1970s, but rather has increased. However, there has not been any increase in the incidence of severely multi-handicapped children. Because of the concomitant decrease in perinatal mortality a considerable net 'gain' in the number of lives saved without cerebral palsy has been achieved."

This situation has been attained in Sweden only by the convergence of multiple favorable medical, economic, and social factors. There are few places in the world where the level of mortality is so low that the negative effects of intensive care can be seen on the population. But this is a specific situation and must not be generalized, even though this trend was recently confirmed by Hagberg [36].

There are so many biases of interpretation [37] that it is not surprising to see such divergent conclusions. An example of the many traps that the epidemiologist must guard against occurred when the public transport system for newborns in New York City was initially organized in the years 1970–1971. Apparently the creation of a specific system for the transport of low birth weight (LBW) premature infants led to a peak in mortality of these babies in the intensive care units. This paradoxical and anecdotal phenomenon was simply a reflection of the change in the way these LBW premature infants were managed in the delivery room: since they now had the possibility of transport, the delivery room personnel resuscitated all infants—even those who previously would have been judged to be beyond saving and would have died without any question of transport. After a short period of apparently unfavorable results, there followed transports that were well planned and organized; also, when possible the woman in labor is transported to a well-equipped medical center prior to delivery.

Another trap to which the epidemiologist is vulnerable lies in the

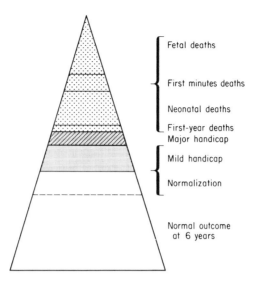

Fig. 1-2 Representation of mortality and morbidity from life *in utero* up to school age.

definition of neonatal mortality. Intensive care often only delays the death of very small premature infants from the first days to the first weeks. Therefore, early neonatal death (i.e., between birth and 7 days) no longer has the same significance. Late neonatal death (≤28 days) is also not satisfactory. Defining mortality on the basis of deaths that occur prior to discharge from intensive care is an improvement, but this concept still neglects several important factors. In addition, there are a significant number of secondary neonatal deaths, that is, those that occur during the first year of life in infants who have been discharged with pulmonary or cerebral disorders or those who are simply at greater risk of sudden death.

It will be important to have statistics on the number of infants at age 1 year who have permanent sequelae of perinatal disorders and those who have transient neuromotor anomalies, because this will give a good idea of their outcome at school age (see below).

The overall significance of these data can be represented by a pyramid as in Figure 1-2. (No attempt has been made at an accurate scale; the intent is simply to provide an illustration of the technique.) Ideally the obstetrician would be given such a pyramid, with percentages noted, for each major gestational pathological condition. Although this is not likely in the near future, it is a reasonable goal.

Conclusions: Proposal for Optimal Follow-up Care of Infants

All newborns should be evaluated based on the following guidelines:

1. All newborns who have had perinatal problems have the right to a convalescence during their first months. During this period of convalescence only the positive aspects of the immediate development should be considered significant to the parents, no matter what anomalies are observed.
2. The same services are offered to all newborns without preselection, since the neonatal period is not always marked by pathological events. The surveillance will be gradually relaxed in all the favorable cases. Physiotherapy and stimulation are indicated for those infants who remain suspect for handicap.
3. Multidisciplinary follow-up is available when necessary, including psychological, neuropediatric, orthopedic, and physiotherapy. There must also be sensorial evaluation, follow-up transfontanellar ultrasound, and EEGs.
4. Early and effective intervention is provided for infants with cerebral motor deficits, without a break between birth and the definitive diagnosis.
5. Continuous care is given to the infant and the family each time transient anomalies of any kind are noted during the first year. Support can then be offered in the areas of psychomotor, sensorial, or language functions, thus lessening the possibility that problems will develop at school age.

References

[1] Treisser A. and Sureau C. Moyens actuels de surveillance du foetus, le concept de souffrance foetale chronique. *Rev. Prat.*, *31*, 329, 1981.
[2] Boisselier P., Lebrun F., Amiel-Tison C. and Sureau C. Arguments en faveur d'une naissance prématurée chez un foetus hypotrophique de mère hypertendue. *Méd. Hyg.*, *39*, 2086, 1981.
[3] Philip A. G. S., Little G. A., Polivy D. R. and Lucey J. F. Neonatal mortality risk for the eighties: the importance of birth weight/gestational age groups. *Pediatrics*, *68*, 122, 1981.
[4] Fancourt R., Campbell S., Harvey D. and Norman A. P. Follow-up study of small-for-dates babies. *Brit. Med. J.*, *1*, 1435, 1976.
[5] Harvey D., Prince J., Bunton J., Parkinson C. and Campbell S. Abilities of children who were small-for-gestational-age babies. *Pediatrics*, *69*, 296, 1982.
[6] Koops B. L., Morgan L. J. and Battaglia F. C. Neonatal mortality risk in

relation to birth weight and gestational age: update. *J. Pediatr.*, *101*, 969, 1982.

[7] Knobloch H., Maloine A., Ellison P. H., Stevens F. and Zdeb M. Considerations in evaluating changes in outcome for infants weighing less than 1,501 grams. *Pediatrics*, *69*, 285, 1982.

[8] Britton S. B., Fitzhardinge P. M. and Ashby S. Is intensive care justified for infants weighing less than 801 grams at birth? *J. Pediatr.*, *99*, 937, 1981.

[9] Hirata T., Epcar J. T., Walsh A., Mednick, J., Harris, M., McGinnis, M. S., Sehring, S. and Papedo, G. Survival and outcome of infants 501 to 750 gm: a six-year experience. *J. Pediatr.*, *102*, 741, 1983.

[10] Green M. and Solnit A. J. Reactions to the threatened loss of a child: a vulnerable child syndrome. *Pediatrics*, *34*, 58, 1964.

[11] Kennel J. H. and Klaus M. H. Care of the mother of the high risk infant. *Clin. Obstet. Gynecol.*, *14*, 926, 1971.

[12] Bentovim A. Emotional disturbances of handicapped pre-school children and their families—attitudes to the child. *Brit. Med. J.*, *2*, 579, 1972.

[13] McCormick M. C., Shapiro S. and Starfield B. Factors associated with maternal opinion of infant development. Clues to the vulnerable child? *Pediatrics*, *69*, 537, 1982.

[14] Hornych H. and Amiel-Tison C. Rétention hydrosaline chez les enfants de faible poids de naissance. *Arch. Fr. Pédiatr.*, *34*, 206, 1977.

[15] Amiel-Tison C., Korobkin R, Hornych H. and Dalisson C. Delayed intracranial hypertension in the premature neonate, following chronic fetal distress. In: *Intensive care in the newborn III*, L. Stern *et al.* (Eds.), p. 239, Masson, New York, 1981.

[16] Grenier A. Diagnostic précoce de l'infirmité motrice cérébrale . . . pour quoi faire? *Ann. Pédiatr.*, *29*, 509, 1982.

[17] Amiel-Tison C. Neurologic evaluation of the small neonate: the importance of head straightening reactions. In: *Modern Perinatal Medicine*, L. Gluck (Ed.), pp. 347–357, Year Book Medical Publishers, Chicago, 1974.

[18] Gross S. J., Oehler J. M. and Eckerman C. O. Head growth and developmental outcome in very low birth weight infants. *Pediatrics*, *71*, 70, 1983.

[19] Hack M., Mostow A. and Miranda S. B. Development of attention in preterm infants. *Pediatrics*, *58*, 669, 1976.

[20] Kutzberg D., Vaughan H. G., Daum C., Grellong B. A., Albin S. and Rotkin L. Neurobehavioral performance of low birth weight infants at 40 weeks conceptional age: comparison with normal fullterm. *Dev. Med. Child Neurol.*, *21*, 590, 1979.

[21] Hunt J. V. Personal communication.

[22] Stewart A. L., Thorburn R. J., Hope P. L., Costello A. M. Del, Goldsmith M., Swain P. and Reynolds E. O. R. Prediction of neurodevelopmental status at 18 months of age by ultrasound and neurological examination. *Abstr. Eur. Soc. Pediatric Res.* 1983.

[23] Stewart, A. Assessment of preterm infant and prognosis. In: *Preterm la-*

bour and its consequences, R. Beard and F. Sharp (Eds.), (pp. 25–36. Royal College of Obstetricians and Surgeons Publ., London, 1985.

[24] Amiel-Tison C., Barrier G., Shnider S. M., Levinson G., Hughes S. C. and Stefani S. J. A new neurologic and adaptative capacity scoring system for evaluating obstetric medications in fullterm newborns. *J. Anesthesiol.*, *56*, 340, 1982.

[25] St. James-Roberts I. Neurological plasticity, recovery from brain insult, and child development. In: *Advances in child development and behavior*, H. W. Reese and L. P. Lipsitt (Eds.), vol. 14, p. 253. Academic Press, New York, 1979.

[26] Kulakowski S. and Larroche J. C. Cranial computerized tomography in cerebral palsy. An attempt at anatomo-clinical and radiological correlations. *Neuropediatrics*, *11*, 339, 1980.

[27] Rutter M. Syndromes attributed to "minimal brain dysfunction" in childhood. *Am. J. Psychiatry*, *139*, 21, 1982.

[28] Gillberg C. and Rasmussen P. Perceptual, motor and additional deficits in seven-year-old children: background factors. *Dev. Med. Child Neurol.*, *24*, 752, 1982.

[29] Rutter M. Psychological sequelae of brain damage in children. *Am. J. Psychiatry*, *138*, 1533, 1981.

[30] Fitzhardinge P. M. and Steven E. M. The small for dates infant. II. Neurological and intellectual sequelae. *Pediatrics*, *50*, 1972.

[31] Kiely J. L., Paneth H. N., Stein Z. and Susser M. Cerebral palsy and newborn care. I. Secular trends in cerebral palsy. *Dev. Med. Child Neurol.*, *23*, 533, 1981.

[32] Kiely J. N., Paneth H. N. Stein Z. and Susser M. Cerebral palsy and newborn care. II. Mortality and neurological impairment in low-birth-weight infants. *Dev. Med. Child Neurol.*, *23*, 650, 1981.

[33] Kiely J. N., Paneth H. N. Stein Z. and Susser M. Cerebral palsy and newborn care. III. Estimated prevalence rates of cerebral palsy under differing rates of mortality and impairment of low-birth-weight infants. *Dev. Med. Child Neurol.*, *23*, 801, 1981.

[34] Stewart A. L., Reynolds E. O. R. and Lipscomb A. P. Outcome for infants of very low birth weight, survey of world literature. *Lancet*, *1*, 1038, 1981.

[35] Hagberg B., Hagberg G. and Olow I. Gains and hazards of intensive neonatal care: an analysis from Swedish cerebral palsy epidemiology. *Dev. Med. Child Neurol.*, *24*, 13, 1982.

[36] Hagberg B., Hagberg G. and Olow I. The changing panorama of cerebral palsy in Sweden. *Acta Paediatr. Scand.*, *73*, 433, 1984.

[37] Pharagh P. and Alberman E. Mortality of low birth weight infants in England and Wales 1953 to 1979. *Arch. Dis. Child.*, *56*, 86, 1981.

2

THE NEUROLOGICAL EVALUATION IN THE NEONATAL PERIOD

Cerebral maturation occurs very rapidly between 28 and 40 weeks of gestation, and therefore the clinical criteria of normalcy must change with the same speed. The level of competence of a full-term newborn or a premature infant having reached the age of term must be evaluated as completely as possible to affirm normal function. We analyze how to carry out this evaluation in the first part of this chapter.

If a pathological condition exists during the first weeks of life, complementary examinations will be more important than the clinical examination; this process is discussed in the second part of this chapter. It is not possible to do a clinical neurological evaluation on the very small premature who is intubated at birth; perhaps a free arm or leg will permit the examiner to evaluate passive tone, but passive tone may also have been affected by the baby's position *in utero*. In addition, the norms of performance before 28 weeks gestational age (GA) have not been established. The norms were established for babies after 28 weeks GA in the mid-1950s on a small group of newborns who represented a very specific part of this population: those who survived without pulmonary disease and for whom GA was not verified by early fetal ultrasound. Because of the lack of norms and because of technical difficulties in the clinical examination, the neurological investigation tends to be put off until after the acute period of the first days of life. During this initial period it is the complementary examinations that provide the essential data; repeated transfontanellar ultrasound, EEG, and fontanometry are widely used.

Later, when the infant is no longer receiving assisted ventilation and when his nutrition is satisfactory, the neurological examination will be progressively completed. It begins with an evaluation of tone, reflexes, and state of consciousness, and later includes demonstration of sensorial function including vision, hearing, contact, and interaction with the environment.

With the passage of time more and more can be learned from the clinical examination. On discharge the infant leaves behind a huge medical chart. How should the observations and results of the examinations over the first weeks or months of life be used in the overall neurological evaluation? They should form a basis for the subsequent follow-up of the child, and should not be communicated to the parents but should remain confidential.

Analysis of Development from 28 to 40 Weeks of Gestation

The order used in this analysis represents only a separation of the different elements of the examination and not a hierarchy. Muscle tone is studied for several reasons: (1) it remains the speciality of the French school of neonatal neurology and (2) it is essential to the expression of the primary reflexes. Technical precision is necessary in each maneuver. (Most technical descriptions are given in the next chapter.) The description of the stages of maturation is from the works of Saint-Anne-Dargassies [1,2]. The choice of maneuvers, their graphic representation, and the different stages of active tone of the neck is from the work of one of us [3,4].

Following the discussion of tone, we cover the primary reflexes, the states of sleep and wakefulness, sensorial abilities, and finally craniocerebral development. Several comments on the maturative levels and the competence of the newborn end the first part of this chapter.

MUSCLE TONE

General thoughts and definitions

Even though neurological study since the mid-1950s has added a great amount of new information to the understanding of muscle tone, we consider that the aspects of the clinical examination of tone described by André Thomas remain essential to the clinical analysis. Therefore this discussion retains the terminology used in the collaboration of Thomas and de Ajuriaguerra [5], and that used by Thomas himself [2,6,7].

PASSIVE TONE.   The analysis of passive tone involves the study of

extensibility and of flapping. *Extensibility* of muscles is observed segment by segment, by a number of maneuvers evaluating the amplitude
of a slow movement executed by the observer with the infant remaining passive. The result can usually be expressed as an angle estimated
by the observer but not measured; alternatively, the result may be
expressed by association with certain anatomical landmarks (the scarf
sign, lateral rotation of the head) or possibly by the gross estimation of
an incurvation (e.g., of the trunk). In all these maneuvers the examiner
must control the force applied and find the infant's limit of function
without creating discomfort.

The study of *flapping* is the evaluation of the amplitude of movement secondary to passive, but rapid, mobilization of a distal segment,
thereby stimulating a braking action by the antagonists. This is most
useful to demonstrate asymmetry of the extremities and also to obtain
the muscle relaxation preliminary to the evaluation of active tone.

ACTIVE TONE.   This is the ability of the infant to respond to everything other than muscle stretching, which explores passive tone. In
other words all that sets in motion *postural and motor activity* is involved in the description of active tone. It is therefore impossible to
consider active tone as one entity (as opposed to passive tone) and to
give an overall description.

1. *Tone "at rest" is used in its usual clinical definition.* It does not
seem useful to debate the existence of tone at rest or the neuro-
physiological definition of resting tone. What is important to us is the
approach to *abnormal tone*, whether it is insufficient or excessive. As
a rule it is unavoidable to use the terms "hypertonic" and "hypotonic"
in international language, despite the imprecision and confusion that
may accompany these terms. In using these terms, therefore, we remain aware of the difficulties inherent in their use.

2. *Postural maintenance is distinct from locomotion.* Classically there
are two different types of performance: (a) *postural aptitude*, which is
involved in head control at all ages, in sitting and standing, as opposed
to (b) *locomotion*, which involves all types of displacement from the
prewalking stage until the acquisition of walking [8–10].

3. *Stimulation of active tone can be under the control of the infant
or the examiner.* Active tone determines spontaneous activity when
controlled by the infant himself, but such activity can be controlled by
the examiner. By stimulating the infant in specific ways while maintaining good contact, the examiner can encourage specific responses
like those we study below in the complementary neuromotor exami-

nation. The postural reflexes described by Vojta [11] and used by some teams are defined as "the aptitude to adapt to changes in position of the body in space" with stereotypical responses evolving from birth until the acquisition of walking. This work was the basis of all the tests that followed. One of us has followed the same line of research in describing the specifically defined conditions that will evoke specific motor actions (12–14).

4. *Anterior–posterior and lateral reactivity.* All the descriptions of active tone and postural activity essentially involve reactivity in the anteroposterior plane. However, one of us (A.G.) has explored lateral reactivity, which is quite significant. It is a more complex function and therefore has greater predictive value when there is early demonstration that it is intact.

Evolution of passive tone with gestational age

Passive tone evolves from global hypotonia (of the axis and extremities) at 28 weeks to a hypertonia of the upper and lower extremities (in flexion) and a strengthening of the flexors and extensors of the axis at 40 weeks. Figure 2-1 describes this progression at intervals of 2 weeks based on six maneuvers or observations: the posture in dorsal decubitus, the heel–ear maneuver, the popliteal angle, the angle of dorsiflexion of the foot, the scarf sign, and the return to flexion of the forearm.

It is possible to separate this evolution into separate stages according to GA because of the gradual acquisition of flexor tone in the caudocephalic direction.

Evolution of active tone with gestational age

This is the most interesting part of the examination. The different stages are partially defined by the strengthening of active tone in the caudocephalic direction. There is also the progressive equalization of the tone of the extensors and flexors of the axis; the anterior muscles (flexors) become stronger slightly later than the posterior muscles (extensors), until their actions are equal at the GA of 38 to 40 weeks.

Figure 2-2 describes this progression at intervals of 2 weeks analyzing four actions: standing posture, passage from lying position to sitting position, return back from sitting to lying, and response to traction using the grasping reflex (see Table 2-1).

The study of active tone necessitates complete freedom of execution by the infant and by the examiner. A good understanding of the responses to be elicited is essential. The infant is placed in a precise position and the response is observed. In the case of analysis of active

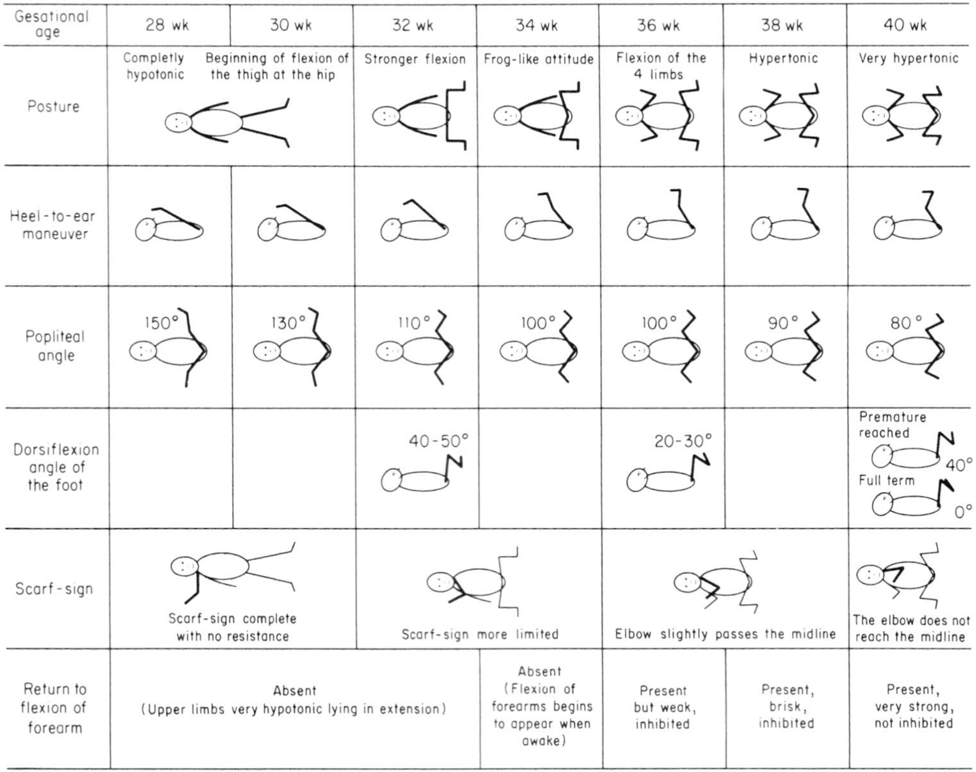

Gestational age	28 wk	30 wk	32 wk	34 wk	36 wk	38 wk	40 wk
Posture	Completely hypotonic	Beginning of flexion of the thigh at the hip	Stronger flexion	Frog-like attitude	Flexion of the 4 limbs	Hypertonic	Very hypertonic
Heel-to-ear maneuver							
Popliteal angle	150°	130°	110°	100°	100°	90°	80°
Dorsiflexion angle of the foot			40-50°		20-30°		Premature reached 40° / Full term 0°
Scarf-sign	Scarf-sign complete with no resistance	Absent (Upper limbs very hypotonic lying in extension)	Scarf-sign more limited		Elbow slightly passes the midline	Elbow slightly passes the midline	The elbow does not reach the midline
Return to flexion of forearm				Absent (Flexion of forearms begins to appear when awake)	Present but weak, inhibited	Present, brisk, inhibited	Present, very strong, not inhibited

Fig. 2-1 Posture and passive tone from 28 to 40 weeks GA.
(From Amiel-Tison C. In: *Pediatrics 16*. A. M. Rudolph (Ed.), 16th ed. Appleton-Century-Crofts, New York, 1977, with permission.)

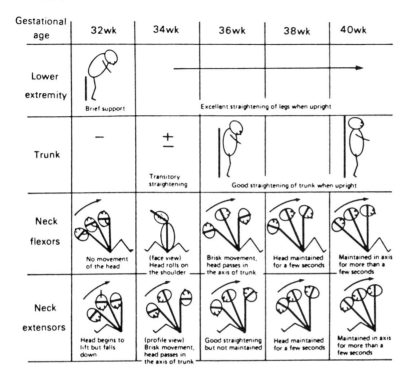

Gestational age	32wk	34wk	36wk	38wk	40wk
Lower extremity	Brief support	Excellent straightening of legs when upright			
Trunk	−	± Transitory straightening	Good straightening of trunk when upright		
Neck flexors	No movement of the head	(face view) Head rolls on the shoulder	Brisk movement, head passes in the axis of trunk	Head maintained for a few seconds	Maintained in axis for more than a few seconds
Neck extensors	Head begins to lift but falls down	(profile view) Brisk movement, head passes in the axis of trunk	Good straightening but not maintained	Head maintained for a few seconds	Maintained in axis for more than a few seconds

Fig. 2-2   Active tone from 32 to 40 weeks gestational age.
(From Amiel-Tison C. In: *Pediatrics 16*, A. M. Rudolph (Ed.), 16th ed.
Appleton-Century-Crofts, New York, 1977, with permission.)

muscle tone of the neck and shoulders, however, the posture of the
newborn is changed, with the speed of this change representing a stimulus to which the infant will react. If the movement is executed too
slowly, the reaction may not be elicited and this lack of response may
be incorrectly interpreted; if the movement is executed too quickly the
active reaction may not be possible, and a simple passive movement of
the head may, for example, be confused with a normal reaction.

Conclusions

It must be emphasized that the analysis of muscle tone and its progression in the premature infant is a field of study almost exclusively
French. Neutral or dissenting opinions are often expressed, like those
of Volpe [15], who feels that in his hands the analysis of passive tone
does not add to the evaluation of maturation. Prechtl [16] does not find

the caudocephalic progression in posture from 28 to 37 weeks. Others like Milani-Comparetti [17] feel that motor organization is more meaningful than tone, which he considers the poorest indicator of maturation.

We feel, on the contrary, that tone is an excellent marker of maturation if it is analyzed with precise technique. The evaluation of passive tone has been wrongly overvalued in the maturation scores [18,19], because this is the easiest part of the examination and can be readily scored in terms of angles. It would seem that an untrained technician can do this evaluation. On the other hand, the evaluation of active tone is often neglected for the opposite reasons: it is the most difficult part of the examination and lends itself least to a numerical score. Both the difficulty and the great interest in this part of the examination stem from the fact that it is the newborn's participation that affects all of his responses.

The neurological examination must not bore the newborn. He must be in communication with the observer. The newborn and the examiner are like two actors on the stage, drawing as much as possible from one another. Routine, boredom, indifference, or the sole interest of arriving at a score—all decrease the value of the neurological evaluation. This does not exclude rigorous observation; the responses to be obtained during the examination must be well understood. The newborn must understand what is being asked of him, and the observer must create the precise situations to obtain specific results. To be of the greatest value the scenario must have meaning for both the players and the audience.

It is indispensable from a conceptual point of view to describe a homogeneous level of maturation, that is, a *cluster of responses* for a given age. Sometimes the responses are very scattered, in which case it is wise to postpone conclusions and to reevaluate at a later time. Adding up numbers and arriving at a score at any price is only of interest to the technical staff and the epidemiologists; it gives nothing of significance to the obstetrician or pediatrician. Finally, it must be noted that early fetal ultrasound is superior to the neurological evaluation for accurate judgment of GA. There is no clinical method that is superior to the 3-day margin of error of fetal ultrasound done before 12 weeks GA, but the clinical knowledge of maturation levels is of fundamental interest. The knowledge of normal responses at different GAs allows for the detection of anomalies. This knowledge is the only semiology that currently exists for the premature infant.

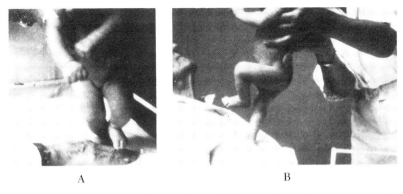

A   B

Fig. 2-3   The automatic walking reflex. (A) While walking the newborn reaches
an obstacle, which is the hand of André Thomas. He adapts his steps and walks
over the obstacle. (B) The newborn walks on an ascending incline formed by
the chest of André Thomas.
(Photos reprinted with permission from Thomas A. and Autgaerden S. "Locomotion from Pre to Postnatal Life," *Clinics in Developmental Medicine*, no.
24, Heinemann, London, 1966.)

THE PRIMARY REFLEXES

The primary reflexes are truly fascinating to observers. The walking
reflex is the one best known to parents and also the reflex that has
been written about most abundantly, particularly by André Thomas
[20]. This fascination for the walking reflex is undoubtedly explained
by the clear demonstration of programming already present in the tiny
fetus. Moreover, it is easy to show that this programming, this primary
automatism, can be modified depending on the circumstances. The films
by André Thomas demonstrating bypassing an obstacle (Fig. 2-3A) or
walking up an incline (Fig. 2-3B) show a sophisticated level of adaptation in the full-term newborn.

Aside from the emotional responses and the minutely detailed descriptions, what is the clinical significance of the study of the primary
reflexes?

Evaluating maturation

Between 28 and 40 weeks the primary reflexes provide little information, as they appear very early and are perfected along with the response capacities of the infant, that is, as active tone evolves. There is
no easy distinction between the Moro reflex at 32 or 34 weeks. The

Table 2-1 Strength of Six Reflexes for Infants between 28 and 40 Weeks' Gestational Age

	28	30	32	34	36	38	40
Sucking reflex	Weak and not really synchronized with deglutition		Stronger and better synchronized with deglutition		Perfect		
Grasping reflex	Present but weak			Stronger		Excellent	
Response to traction	Absent		Begins to appear	Strong enough to lift part of the body weight		Strong enough to lift all of the body weight	
Moro reflex	Weak, obtained just once, incomplete		Complete reflex —————→		————→		
Crossed extension	Flexion and extension in a random pattern, purposeless reaction		Good extension but no tendency to adduction		Tendency to adduction but imperfect	Complete response with extension, adduction, fanning of the toes	
Automatic walking		—	Pretty good. Very fast Tiptoeing. Begins tiptoeing with good support on the sole and a righting reaction of the legs for a few seconds			A premature who has reached 40 weeks walks in a toe–heel progression or tiptoes. A full-term newborn of 40 weeks walks in a heel–toe progression on the whole sole of the foot.	

Source: From C. Amiel-Tison, in *Pediatrics 16*, A. M. Rudolph (Ed.), 16th ed. Appleton-Century-Crofts, New York, 1977, with permission.

same is true for sucking and swallowing: the reflex exists very early, since the fetus swallows *in utero*. However, the healthy newborn can only provide his own nutrition from 34 weeks GA. This is the reason that Table 2-1 is less precise than Figures 2-1 and 2-2; it shows tendencies rather than stages. Some of the most current findings are represented: sucking and swallowing, grasping with the fingers, the Moro reflex, and walking. The response to traction, which is the complement of grasping with the fingers, is an excellent maneuver for evaluating active tone.

The crossed extension reflex is particularly useful in evaluating maturation, since one of the components, adduction, begins to appear at 35 to 36 weeks and is complete at 38 to 40 weeks. Once the reflex is complete at the age of term, there is nothing further to be learned from it. The technical description of the evaluation of this reflex is therefore included here, since it is not included in subsequent neurological evaluations during the first year.

CROSSED EXTENSION.   One foot is stimulated by rubbing the plantar surface with the lower extremity held in extension. The threefold response is observed in the other lower extremity: (1) extension after a

Fig. 2-4   The crossed extension reflex. The free leg reacts with extension, fanning of the toes, and adduction, which bring the free foot to the foot that was stimulated.

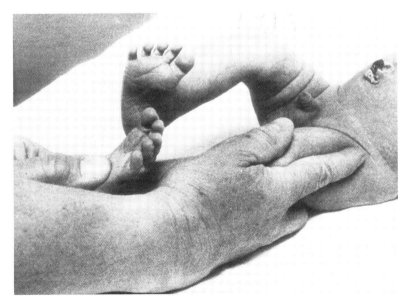

rapid movement of withdrawal in flexion, (2) fanning of the toes, and (3) adduction, bringing the foot toward the foot which was stimulated. The first two parts of the response are constant; it is the adduction that is dependent on maturation. Adduction is slight at 36 weeks and perfect at 40 weeks (Fig. 2-4).

Evaluating normal cerebral function

The primary reflexes are part of the normal behavior of the premature and full-term newborn. The sucking and swallowing reflex allows him to take nourishment and must be coordinated and perfect, whereas the Moro and grasping reflexes can be seen in the opposite way, as a hindrance to voluntary motor activity (seen below). This automatic "parasitical" motor activity stimulated by the slightest abrupt movement of the neck or the slightest touch is a nuisance that the newborn retains until a subsequent stage of maturation when inhibitory brain function begins.

Thus the purpose of testing several of the primary reflexes during the neurological examination is to look for cerebral dysfunction. The interpretation necessarily evolves over the course of several months.

For the premature or full-term newborn in whom cerebral abnormality is suspected, the presence of brisk, reproducible primary reflexes that are easy to elicit is a good sign; weak or absent reflexes signify CNS depression, usually associated with a decreased level of consciousness and hypotonia. A brief philosophy of the primary reflexes in the first weeks of life can be summarized: "to have or have not."

During the first months of life it is to be hoped that the infant's primary reflexes are difficult to elicit or have disappeared, since their disappearance demonstrates higher cerebral control. The age limits for the disappearance of each reflex vary widely. The infant should be regarded as a whole, and pathological significance should only be attributed to those cases where there is clear and global delay in the disappearance of primary reactivity.

A philosophical digression

A practical justification for the Moro and grasping reflexes has been proposed. The gripping of the fingers can be seen as reinforcing the hold of simian babies clutching their mothers' breast without any other means of support. See the situation illustrated in Figure 2-5.

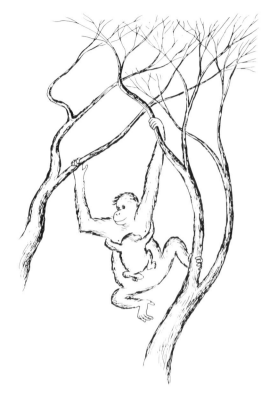

Fig. 2-5 The Moro and grasping reflexes, first seen in our cousins who live
in the trees.
(Reprinted with permission from Amiel-Tison C. and Grenier A. *Est-ce ainsi
que les enfants naissent?* Robert Laffont, Paris, 1983.)

THE STATES OF SLEEP AND WAKEFULNESS

The general behavior of a newborn during the 10-minute neurological
examination is a significant part of the overall evaluation. The predom-
inant state of consciousness is noted, whether normal, lethargic, or
hyperexcitable. The change from one state to another—toward wakefulness of toward sleep—may be noted, and the communication with
surroundings during a calm period of wakefulness is noted. For the
full-term infant the normal sleep–wakefulness pattern is taught to
mothers so that they can better understand and respond to this rhythm:
asleep for 50 minutes, awake for ~10 minutes. These periods will
lengthen gradually until the sleep period is ~2 hours and wakefulness

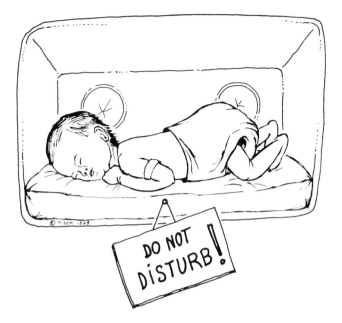

Fig. 2-6 The sleeping state of the convalescent newborn must be as well protected as possible.
(Reprinted from Amiel-Tison C. and Lebrun F. *ABC de Médecine Néonatale*, Masson, Paris, 1980, with permission.)

can reach 20–30 minutes. It is just as important that doctors and nurses understand this pattern so that they can respect the periods of sleep as much as possible (Fig. 2-6). In current psychological research, however, it has become important to distinguish the various states of sleep and wakefulness and the passage from one to another. Using behavioral observation and polygraphic studies, several groups have made advances in this area. Prechtl [21] in particular proposes a classification based on four variables that are indicators of the state of sleep or wakefulness: opening of the eyes, breathing, spontaneous motor activity, and vocalization. Five states are defined according to the changes in the four variables (Table 2-2). An interval of observation of 3 minutes is used to describe the various states. This is long enough to ignore momentary instability.

Many aspects of the neurological examination vary with the state of wakefulness. For precise comparisons of neurological function the exact state should be defined and noted for each evaluation. However,

Table 2-2   States of Sleep–Wakefulness

State	Signs
1	Eyes closed, regular respiration, no movements
2	Eyes closed, irregular respiration, no gross movement
3	Eyes open, no gross movements
4	Eyes open, gross movements, no crying
5	Eyes open or closed, crying

Source: After Prechtl H. F. R. and O'Brien M. J. Behavioural states of the full-term newborn. The emergence of a concept. In: *Psychobiology of the human newborn*, P. Stratton (Ed.), pp. 53–69. John Wiley, New York, 1982.

in the intensive care unit or in an office consultation this analytical precision is not practical. The clinician should examine the infant in an optimal state of wakefulness, that is, Prechtl's state 3 or 4. In the event that this state is unattainable, only repeated examinations will determine whether it is merely circumstantial or whether an abnormality is present. Either the infant must be awakened more vigorously, time must be taken to calm him, or the examination must be put off to a future date.

Observing the passage between different states allows evaluation of the infant's interaction with his environment. From the first days of life the infant establishes interaction with his mother by changing states of wakefulness, as seen in Brazelton's study [22,23]. It is also important to observe and note the changes of states during the EEG examination. This provides a component of interpretation in addition to the electromyographic changes in the chin and ocular motility.

In light of recent research on "liberated" motor activity, another variable can be added to those described by Prechtl. That is the intense communication that occurs after manual fixation of the neck during the preparatory period of the examination. During that period transient hand–eye coordination and voluntary motor activity can be observed that is completely different from the spontaneous motor activity observed in the newborn. It is therefore a state different from the five previously described states.

SENSORIAL ABILITIES

The sensorial abilities of the premature and the full-term newborn are considered very important in the evaluation of competence. Recent work has examined the great sensitivity of the entire system and the coordination between each function. Clinically only vision and hearing play a part in the routine evaluation.

Vision

Sensitivity to light exists at birth. The infant placed in front of a window keeps his eyes fixed on the light when his head is turned laterally to the right or left by the examiner. The same test can be done with a penlight. The infant will fix on the light and turn his eyes and head to the right or left to follow the light source.

The newborn cannot accommodate until the age of 3 months. Until that time an object or face must be placed at a distance of ~30 cm (12 in.) to obtain interest and fixation. It is in this way that visual communication is tested. The intense regard that appears to be fixed on the eyes of the observer is called "eye-to-eye contact" and exists in the first days.

Several studies have shown the progression of vision in the premature infant with cerebral maturation. However, the application of this progression in the routine of the neonatal center is difficult. The study of visual following in the premature infant examined in an isolette only became part of the routine clinical examination after the work of Daum *et al.* [24] in 1980. The "bull's-eye" is a round piece of cardboard printed with glossy black and white concentric circles. It is held 20–30 cm (8–12 in.) from the newborn's face; the infant's head is held by the observer with a flat hand to allow for voluntary rotation (Fig. 2-7). When the infant has fixed his gaze on the bull's-eye, it is moved to the right and then to the left; the eyes and then the head follow. It is simple to perform, and the response is easy to evaluate with good interobserver reliability. The work of Daum showed that fixation and following began at 34 weeks GA. Therefore, when the response is positive it is a very good test of normalcy after 34 weeks GA.

Hearing

Sensitivity to sounds exists at birth and even before, as has been shown by recent research on fetal hearing. The evaluation of hearing is part of the neurological examination. Using the voice or a bell, it is easy to obtain a response to the sound in the form of a facial gesture or an orientation toward the source of the sound. Using white noise from an acoustic stimulator is more precise; if the response is hesitant the infant will be retested in the following months.

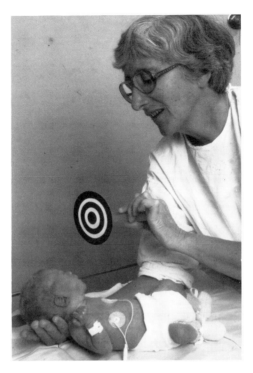

Fig. 2-7   Visual pursuit evaluated in premature infant at 36 weeks GA with a bull's-eye.

CRANIOCEREBRAL DEVELOPMENT

Examination of the head: evolution of head circumference

From the day of birth all through the first year, observation, palpation, and measurements of the head are the primary elements of the neurological examination. The *posterior fontanelle* is the first to close and is usually not palpable after 6 weeks of age. The size of the *anterior fontanelle* is quite variable, as is the date of its closure, which can be between 10 and 20 months. On palpation, disjunction or overriding of sutures will have different significance depending on the infant's age at the time of the examination.

The shape of the head can suggest a *craniosynostosis*. The head is long and narrow in a synostosis of the sagittal sutures; the anterior half of the head is wide and the forehead flat in a synostosis of the coronal

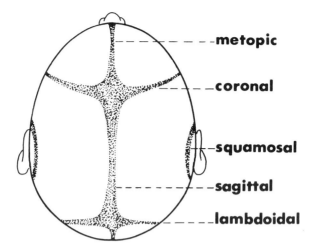

Fig. 2-8   Fontanelles and sutures.

suture. A wide anterior half of the skull with a round forehead suggests hydrocephalus, while a large head with a very prominent occiput suggests a Dandy–Walker malformation.

Measuring the head clinically involves measuring the largest fronto-occipital circumference with a tape measure. It is a simple, reproducible measurement that has been shown to be analogous to the cranial volume measured by sophisticated radiological techniques. The results of the measurement of head circumference are recorded on curves like those reproduced in Figure 3-3 [25].

MATURATIVE LEVELS AND COMPETENCE OF THE NEWBORN: SOME COMMENTS

Neurological maturation and gestational age

The use of the neurological evaluation to determine GA was based on a dogma of a fixed progression of development of the fetal nervous system without regard to the external influences—that is, despite any gestational anomalies. Although this concept can be applied to the majority of fetuses, there are exceptions. Gould *et al.* noted in 1972 [26] that unfavorable intrauterine conditions can accelerate neurological development. One of us [27] confirmed these results on 16 newborns between 30 and 37 weeks GA who showed a neurological maturation at least 4 weeks greater than estimated by accurate dates. Each of these

16 pregnancies was abnormal (maternal hypertension that was permanent or secondary to pregnancy, uterine malformation, or multiple pregnancy). The hypothesis of an increased secretion of corticosteroids by the fetus in response to the repeated stress has been proposed as the stimulus for the advanced maturation. In fact advanced pulmonary maturation is seen in situations where the fetus is under stress and has also been induced by administration of corticosteroids to the pregnant woman. These data show that fetal maturation is programmed but is possibly sensitive to unfavorable conditions. Therefore, retrospective dating of high-risk pregnancies, particularly in cases of maternal hypertension or multiple pregnancies, must be regarded with caution.

Another observation that can be made on these newborns with acceleration of neurological maturation, is that the clinical state at birth and neurological outcome are usually excellent. It seems that prolonged stress that is not intense enough to cause fetal morbidity or mortality can exist without danger to the fetus while accelerating maturation. These observations led to the notion of a threshhold in the consequences of an insult to the fetal brain.

The opposite phenomenon, delayed maturation *in utero*, most likely exists but is harder to demonstrate clinically. This is because, using the parameters of contact and tone, it is difficult to differentiate signs of CNS depression from lag in maturation (a phenomenon seen frequently in infants of diabetic mothers). Other less constructive viewpoints came from misuse of the clinical method described. We will only give a very recent example from the epidemiological work of Rush *et al.* [28]. Nurse practitioners examined 682 newborns, and 19 maneuvers were coded and clustered statistically. The findings were that neurological maturity is more strongly linked to somatic development than to GA. We feel that this is an example of how the distortion of a clinical method can unfortunately lead to inappropriate conclusions.

Apparent fragility of the most recently acquired capacities

Hypotonia of the flexors of the neck and the upper extremities is a frequently observed characteristic of moderate cerebral abnormality of obstetrical origin in the full-term newborn [29]. The repartition of tone in such an infant appears like that which is seen in a normal infant 1 month younger, at 36 weeks GA. However, most often this is of short duration and occurs during the first week of life. The newborn will recover the tone corresponding to his GA of 40 weeks in the same time span as expected for the resolution of circulatory disturbances and edema secondary to the birth process, suggesting a link between the two events.

The hypothesis raised here is that the functions most recently acquired are most fragile, and there are transient returns to the preceding stage of development. It should be noted that as in advance of maturation the existence of a threshold is likely: a moderate attack results in this transient regression that is completely reversible, whereas a more severe attack can result in a cluster of pathological signs linked to true cellular damage that may result in permanent sequelae.

Habituation, a subcortical phenomenon; modulation of habituation, a cortical phenomenon?

Distinguishing between habituation and modulation of habituation helps in understanding the behavior observed in newborns. Demonstrating habituation has been part of the neurological examination of the newborn since the work of Brazelton in 1973 [22]. This phenomenon's significance is based on the fact that habituation is considered evidence of cerebral function that is higher than that of the primary automatisms. Its inclusion in the neurological examination was a reaction to the classical examination that tested reflex behavior in a simplistic and stereotypical way—looking only for the presence or absence of each reaction. Habituation was felt to be a learned skill.

However, recent observers have shown that this ability exists in newborns with anencephaly and hydranencephaly. Thus, it is likely that the subcortical structures are capable of producing such a complex behavior. Therefore, such behavior can no longer be considered in itself in the domain or cortical function. It is difficult to describe this behavior as reflecting cognitive or affective responses implying cortical participation, since habituation and consolability by the voice of the observer have been seen in infants with total absence of the cortex. It seems that certain social behaviors, such as consolability, are part of the primary automatisms in the same way as the smile or the attraction of hand to mouth.

A more qualitative evaluation is probably necessary to test cortical function; such an evaluation would show the ability of the full-term newborn to modify his responses. The goal for the healthy newborn would be to produce a rich variety of nonstereotypical responses to the environment, and by contrast, stereotypical responses would be expected in cases of cerebral dysfunction. It is therefore in the evaluation of contact and of interaction that the newborn can be shown to be "intact." It is in the plasticity of his behavior that his "competence" must be found [30].

In the same spirit, the modification of the sleep–wakefulness states takes on greater significance: "The variability of state indicates the infant's capacities for self-organization" [23].

Imitation, intermodal coordination, and representation in the newborn

In 1977, using rigorous experimental conditions, Meltzoff demonstrated the capacity of an infant aged 12–21 days to imitate the facial expressions of an adult he is facing [31]. These observations were met with surprise by pediatricians. Yet it cannot be denied that the newborn will open his mouth, move his tongue, and close his eyes in imitation of the observer. This capacity implies an innate association between what is seen and what is done by the infant himself that is an intermodal coordination that predates experience. Meltzoff recently refuted Piaget's theories of the exclusive role of learning in imitation [32] by demonstrating this ability to imitate in a full-term newborn at age 42 minutes. There are very possibly other innate capacities, and there must be a reevaluation of the theories of social and cognitive development [33]. To understand better when these capacities begin, clinicians must observe the premature infant along these lines. The imitation of facial gestures is not solely an ability of the full-term newborn (see Fig. 2-9).

Fig. 2-9 Imitation of facial expression in a premature newborn at 36 weeks GA.

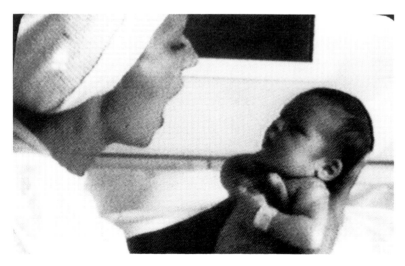

Clinical Signs and Interpretation
of Pathological Findings

The clinician uses the same observations and maneuvers to evaluate maturative level on one hand and on the other hand to verify the absence of abnormality. In the presence of signs or symptoms there must be additional investigations: a brief summary of the type of information that can be obtained from these investigations follows. All the data are assembled in an attempt to define a syndrome or find an etiology.

The clusters of symptoms are summarized. For the premature infant it is those symptoms observed in the intensive care unit and later while recuperating and growing to the age of term. In the full-term newborn it is those symptoms observed during the first weeks of life that are evaluated. However, it is the clinical progression that will be analyzed, not one specific sign. The goal is not to summarize the neonatal cerebral abnormality but to interpret the data, which is the key to subsequent follow-up.

INFORMATION FROM CURRENTLY USED
INVESTIGATION TECHNIQUES

Transillumination is the complement of the first examination of the skull. The use of a simple pocket lamp with pliable border or a more sophisticated lamp with a cold-light source, like a "chun-gun," in a dark room, can show an abnormal diffusion of light in the case of an abnormal fluid collection whether peripheral or intraventricular (in the case when the cerebral coat is of reduced thickness): a subdural collection, cerebral atrophy, porencephaly, or hydrocephaly. The size of an acceptable *halo* depends on the type of light source used. Less than 1 cm is considered normal with a basic electric light. There are established norms, depending on GA, for the chun-gun [34] that exclude unnecessary pathological interpretations. In spite of its advantages, transillumination has been largely replaced by ultrasound when the machine is available.

Auscultation of the skull can provide important diagnostic information. The presence of an intense bruit suggests an arteriovenous malformation.

Most neonatal intensive care units are equipped with a portable *ultrasound* machine that allows for repeated examinations without moving the newborn. The *transfontanellar echogram* is an invaluable examination that is simple and gives results of excellent quality. The indications are wide: all newborns weighing <1500 g and all those who have neurological signs. Repetition of the examination over several weeks gives the ability to follow the evolution, particularly in cases of intracranial hemorrhages. Hemorrhages are very easily visualized; however, errors of interpretation are possible with a very congested choroid plexus or a very dense periventricular germinative zone. The poor quality of the peripheral images make the diagnosis of a subarachnoid hemorrhage uncertain.

Fontanometry gives very reliable figures in the evaluation of ICH [35]. Several instruments are in use that either give a specific measurement or give the results in the form of a curve. Intracranial pressure at rest in a full-term infant is approximately equal to 10 cm (100 mm) of water. A value of 15 cm indicates an increase in pressure; greater values are dangerous and are associated with clinical signs of ICH and the risk of apnea and convulsions.

Electroencephalography (EEG) gives essential data that must be interpreted according to GA, since maturation between 28 and 40 weeks is accompanied by significant EEG changes [36,37]. The anomalies of the neonatal EEG are relatively nonspecific and are often associated with transient metabolic disorders or the administration of anticonvulsant drugs. The tracings must therefore be repeated, and it is the persistence of abnormalities that suggests a specific lesion. The EEG will be done very early, from the first days of life, then repeated several times, at intervals of 1 to 2 weeks. The best clinical correlations are obtained in the acute phase of anoxic ischemic encephalopathy with critical changes, and even better correlation with intercritical changes. Poor prognosis in severe intraventricular hemorrhage in the VLBW infant is best correlated with positive rolandic spikes indicating cellular damage.

The best long-term correlations are obtained in anoxic ischemic encephalopathy in the full-term newborn [38]. On the whole a normal tracing or one that quickly normalizes has a good correlation with a favorable outcome and suggests normalcy similar to normalization in the clinical examination. However, some infants who have no bioelectric abnormality will nonetheless develop major sequelae during their first months. It must therefore be realized that certain encephalopathies only affect the subcortical regions, particularly the brain stem, and are mute from the bioelectric point of view. These lesions should be identifiable using brain stem evoked potentials.

CLUSTERS OF SYMPTOMS

CNS depression

This cluster of signs involves defects in three areas: consciousness, tone, and primary reflexes. Different degrees of lethargy and hyporeactivity are observed, from inability to obtain a correct state of wakefulness and some interaction, to complete coma. There is little spontaneous activity and crying is rare. The tone is globally deficient, with global hypotonia at rest and in the maneuvers evaluating active tone. Sometimes an abnormality of tone can be localized, most commonly to the upper part of the body. Either the primary reflexes are totally absent, or they are difficult to obtain on repeated attempts and incomplete. In particular, deficient sucking and swallowing can make feeding dangerous or impossible.

It is important to repeat the examination to determine whether these signs are permanent or variable, which helps in the understanding of etiology. Signs that are fixed, varying little from one day to another, are often associated with a variety of prenatal causes. Variable signs usually worsen over the first few days, followed by improvement; they are usually seen with recent distress, often as a result of the birth process itself.

Hyperexcitability and convulsions

Hyperexcitability is often difficult to define as abnormal, since the full-term newborn is often irritable during the first days of life. Tremulousness and clonus, episodes of inconsolable crying, excessive sensitivity to light and noise, and spontaneous Moro reflexes can be seen. Sometimes these are definitely pathological with clonus of all four extremities, insufficient sleep, high-pitched cry, and global hypertonia.

Convulsions may accompany this hyperexcitability. They are usually overt, with focal or multifocal clonus. They are generally overdiagnosed rather than underdiagnosed. The converse is true for the convulsions that are seen with the previously described signs of CNS depression. These convulsions are most frequently subtle and localized to one muscle group. They are erratic and are often missed clinically. When the convulsions are repeated at very brief intervals, the state of consciousness worsens, and coma ensues, this is *status epilepticus*. The EEG is indispensable in the identification of convulsive states in the newborn; however, treatment can be instituted based on a suggestive clinical examination.

Intracranial hypertension

Intracranial pressure can be elevated in many pathological conditions in the neonatal period. The diagnosis is based on a cluster of cranial and neurological signs. The cranial signs are described below (see Chapter 3), particularly the importance of disjunction of the squamous sutures. The maturation of the skull plays a role in the respective importance of suture disjunction versus neurological signs.

The neurological signs are specific in their grouping: lethargy, vomiting, yawning, irregular respiration, apneic episodes, bradycardia, and ocular signs—particularly the sunset sign, either intermittent or persistent. The problems of axial tone that precede or accompany these signs are themselves very specific. The technique of evaluating axial tone is described below (see Chapter 3). All the aspects of hypertonia of the posterior muscles can be seen in ICH, from simple imbalance of passive axial tone to significant opisthotonos with the inability of the head to fall forward while in the sitting position.

This symptom cluster must be recognized early, so that a palliative treatment can be started and an investigation into the exact cause of the ICH can begin.

CLINICAL GRADATION OF THE FULL-TERM NEWBORN

Clinical signs are more easily recognized in the full-term newborn than in the premature newborn. An evident grouping of symptoms allows a simple classification at the end of the first week. The choice of 1 week was made because in France the usual length of the postnatal hospitalization has classically been 6–7 days and, more importantly, it is our experience that this is the time period that corresponds to the disappearance of most minor neurological signs linked to the birth process. A gradation in three levels (Table 2-3) is used for the neurological ob-

Table 2-3 Gradation of Signs of Cerebral Distress for the Full-Term Newborn during the Neonatal Period

Level of distress	Signs and symptoms
Mild	Abnormalities of tone and hyperexcitability (seizures excluded)
Moderate	Same signs as mild form plus signs of CNS depression and possibly signs of ICH (isolated seizures included)
Severe	Repeated seizures and overt CNS depression

servation done on day 7 and results in good correlation with long-term outcome.

ETIOLOGICAL ORIENTATION

When the etiology of cerebral damage is not evident, everything must be done to discover the cause, including (1) analysis of the gestational events, (2) reevaluation of fetal monitoring, (3) reinvestigation of maternal drugs and family history, (4) study of the labor and delivery, including interviewing the labor team as soon as possible after delivery and later reconstructing the events, (5) examination of the evolutive or static character of the neurological signs, (6) study of any CT scan data (CT scan should have been done within the first 3 days in the case of significant but unexplained distress), and (7) later a karyotype and more specific research if the etiology is still unknown.

Several empirical observations emerge from our experience in the analysis of etiology of cerebral distress in full-term newborns:

1. The cause remains unknown in a high proportion of cases (approximately one-third) and therefore can escape thorough evaluation done in the best conditions of communication between obstetrician and pediatrician.
2. Obstetrical risk factors that did not cause neurological signs during the first week of life should not be held responsible for any future problems. Thus it is reaffirmed that the full-term newborn always expresses signs and symptoms of cerebral dysfunction, even if they are benign and transient.
3. The number of cases of perinatal cerebral damage have universally decreased and have become rare in well-staffed and well-equipped maternity centers. In recent years the cause of damage has moved from the obstetrical to the gestational domain, in particular fetal circulatory accidents that may be silent or undetectable during fetal life using techniques currently available.

In conclusion, this schematic classification of clinical signs is admittedly oversimplified and is not entirely in line with reality. The variability of risk factors and symptomatology often leaves the clinician a large margin of interpretation. Nevertheless, this classification includes the most frequently encountered situations and can lead to a therapeutic approach for which there is a general consensus.

References

[1] Saint-Anne-Dargassies S. La maturation neurologique des prématurés. *Etudes néonatales*, 4, 71–122, 1955.

[2] Saint-Anne-Dargassies S. *Le développement neurologique du nouveau-né à terme et prématuré*, 2nd ed. Masson, Paris, 1974.

[3] Amiel-Tison C. Neurological evaluation of the maturity of newborn infants. *Arch. Dis. Child.*, 43, 89–93, 1968.

[4] Amiel-Tison C. Neurological evaluation of the small neonate: the importance of the head straightening reactions. In: *Modern perinatal medicine*, L. Gluck (Ed.), pp. 347–357. Year Book Medical Publishers, Chicago, 1974.

[5] Thomas A. and Ajuriaguerra J. de. *Etude sémiologique du tonus musculaire*. Editions Médicales Flammarion, Paris, 1949.

[6] Thomas A. and Saint-Anne-Dargassies S. *Etudes neurologiques sur le nouveau-né et le jeune nourrisson*. Masson, Paris, 1952.

[7] Stambak M. and Ajuriaguerra J. de. Evolution de l'extensibilité musculaire depuis la naissance jusqu'à l'âge de 2 ans. *Presse Méd.*, 66, 24–36, 1958.

[8] Illingworth R. S. *The development of the infant and young child*, 5th ed., Churchill Livingstone, London, 1972.

[9] Koupernik C. and Dailly R. *Développement neuro-psychique du nourrisson*, 3rd ed. Presses Universitaires de France, Paris, 1976.

[10] Touwen B. Neurological development in infancy. *Clinics in developmental medicine*, no. 58. Spastic International Medical Publications, London, 1976.

[11] Vojta V. *Die cerebralen Bewegungsstörungen in Saüglingsalter*. Fruhdiagnose und Fruhtherapie. F. Enke Verlag, Stuttgart, 1974.

[12] Grenier A. Introduction à la journée d'étude de dépistage et de traitement précoce des Infirmes Moteurs Cérébraux. *Cahiers du Cercle de Documentation et d'Information pour la Rééducation des I.M.C.*, Paris, 52, 5, 1972.

[13] Grenier A., Vima Ph., Solomiac J. and Solomiac J. Examen neuro-moteur complémentaire chez les nourrissons suspects d'I.M.C. *Cahiers du Cercle de Documentation et d'Information pour la Rééducation des I.M.C.*, Paris, 65, 7, 1975.

[14] Grenier A. La Réaction Latérale d'Abduction chez les nourrissons à risque élevé. Société de Neurologie Infantile. *Congrès de Marseille*, 1977.

[15] Volpe J. J. *Neurology of the newborn*, p. 69. Saunders, Philadelphia, 1981.

[16] Prechtl H. F. R., Fargel J. W., Weinmann H. M. and Bakker H. H. Postures, mobility and respiration of low-risk pre-term infants. *Dev. Med. Child Neurol.*, 21, 3–27, 1979.

[17] Milani-Comparetti A. The neurophysiologic and clinical implications of studies on fetal motor behavior. *Semin. Perinatol.*, 5, 183–188, 1981.

[18] Dubowitz L. M., Dubowitz V. and Goldberg C. Clinical assessment of gestational age in the newborn infant. *J. Pediatr.*, 77, 1–10, 1970.

[19] Ballard J. L., Novak K. K. and Driver M. A simplified score for assessment of fetal maturation of newly born infants. *J. Pediatr.*, 95, 769–774, 1979.

[20] Thomas A. and Autgaerden S. *Locomotion from pre to postnatal life*. Clinics in Developmental Medicine, no. 24. Heinemann, London, 1966.

[21] Prechtl H. F. R. and O'Brien M. J. Behavioural states of the full-term newborn. The emergence of a concept. In: *Psychobiology of the human newborn*, P. Stratton (Ed.), pp. 53–69. John Wiley, New York, 1982.

[22] Brazelton T. B. *Neonatal behavioral assessment scale*. London National Spastic Society, London, 1973.

[23] Brazelton T. B. Behavioral competence of the newborn infant. *Sem. Perinatol.*, 3, 35–44, 1979.

[24] Daum C., Kurtzberg D., Ruff H. and Vaughan H. Preterm development of visual and auditory orienting in very low birth weight infants. *Pediatr. Res.*, 14, abst. 41, 1980.

[25] Nelhaus G. Composite international and interracial graphs. *Pediatrics*, 41, 106, 1968.

[26] Gould J. B., Gluck L. and Kulovich M. V. The acceleration of neurological maturation in high stress pregnancy and its relation to fetal lung maturity. *Pediatr. Res.*, 6, 276, 1972.

[27] Amiel-Tison C. Possible acceleration of neurological maturation following high risk pregnancy. *Am. J. Obstet. Gynecol.*, 138, 303–306, 1980.

[28] Rush D., Cassano P., Wilson A. V., Königsberger R. J. and Cohen J. Newborn neurologic maturity relates more strongly to concurrent somatic development than gestational age. *Am. J. Perinatol.*, 1, 12, 1983.

[29] Amiel-Tison C. Pediatric contribution to the present knowledge on the neurobehavioral status of infants at birth. In: *Neonatal cognition: beyond the blooming buzzing confusion*, J. Melher and R. Fox (Eds.), Lawrence Erlbaum, Hillsdale, N. J., 1985, pp. 365–380.

[30] Brazelton T. B. Precursors for the development of emotions in early infancy. In: *Emotion, theory, research and experience*, vol. 2, pp. 35–55. Academic Press, New York, 1983.

[31] Meltzoff A. N. and Moore M. K. Imitation of facial and manual gestures by human neonates. *Science*, 198, 75–78, 1977.

[32] Meltzoff A. N. Imitation, intermodal co-ordination and representation in early infancy. In: *Infancy and epistemology*, G. Butterworth (Ed.). Harvester Press, Brighton, 1981.

[33] Meltzoff A. N. and Moore M. K. The origins of imitation in infancy: paradigm, phenomena, and theories. In: *Advances in infancy research*, L. P. Lippsitt and C. Rovee-Collin (Eds.), vol. 2. Ablex, Norwood N. J., 1983.

[34] Vyhmeister N., Schneider S. and Cha C. Cranial transillumination norms of premature infants. *J. Pediatr.*, 91, 980, 1977.

[35] Philipp A. G. S. Noninvasive monitoring of intracranial pressure. *Clin. Perinatol.*, 6, 123–137, 1979.

[36] Dreyfus-Brisac C. Ontogenesis of the brain bioelectrical activity and sleep organization in neonates and infants. In: *Human growth*, F. Falkner and J. Tanner (Eds.), pp. 397–472. Plenum Press, New York, 1979.

[37] Tharp B. R. Neonatal electroencephalography. In: *Progress in perinatal neurology*, R. Korobkin and C. Guilleminault (Eds.), pp. 31–64. Williams & Wilkins, Baltimore, 1981.

[38] Monod N., Pajot N. and Guidasci S. The neonatal EEG. Statistical studies and prognostic value in full-term and pre-term babies. *Electroencephalogr. Clin. Neurophysiol.*, 7, 302–315, 1977.

3

NORMAL DEVELOPMENT DURING THE FIRST YEAR OF LIFE: Identification of Anomalies and Use of the Grid

Method of Examination

The neurological examination described is a simple, rapid evaluation easily administered and easily integrated into the routine pediatric examination. This method was first published in 1976 [1], and the first results appeared in 1978. [2].

The results of the examination are evaluated most effectively on a grid that takes into account the stage of development (see Appendix). Such a grid has been used for the monthly examinations of infants through the first year of life.

The grid is presented in the logical order of the physical examination. Examination of the skull is accomplished while obtaining the history. Passive tone is evaluated as the infant lies quietly on the examination table. Assessment of active tone and testing the primary and the tendon reflexes follows. The examination concludes with evaluation of postural reactions. Each element of passive tone, active tone, and reflexes is compared with normal development and is grouped according to the normal patterns for each trimester. Any abnormal result is recorded in a hatched area, thereby permitting immediate assessment of the infant's normalcy. Because each maneuver can be evaluated in a simple horizontal perusal, the design permits rapid screening of the grid. This feature is especially useful at the end of the first year. It is preferable that a second person transcribe the results of the examination. This serves two purposes: (1) the examiner is free to devote full attention to the examination, and (2) objectivity is increased, in that the examiner will not be biased by the results of the previous examinations. All examinations are carried out *at corrected age*, thereby permitting assessment of full-term and preterm infants according to the same criteria.

This is not a complete neurological examination, in that it does not include an evaluation of cranial nerves, muscle atrophy or fibrillations, among other factors. As mentioned previously, this is a basic evaluation that can be used as a starting point for further investigation if indicated. The evaluation is not designed to include psychomotor testing and therefore is not expected to uncover abnormalities of behavior, sociability, or fine motor performance.

It is the rapid evolution of active tone during the first year of life that allows for precise landmarks of normal neuromotor development [3–6]. As discussed above, maturation is so rapid between 28 and 40 weeks GA, that it is possible to describe changes by 2-week intervals.

Fig. 3-1 Passive tone in upper and lower extremities. From 28 to 40 weeks GA, muscle tone in flexor muscles increases in caudocephalic progression, as indicated by posture, scarf sign (evaluating extensibility in upper limbs), and popliteal angle (evaluating extensibility in lower limbs). Within the first year of life, muscle tone in flexor muscles decreases in a cephalocaudal progression to reach a global hypotonia maximum at 8 to 10 months.
(From Amiel-Tison C. In: *Neonate cognition*, J. Mehler and R. Fox (Eds.). Lawrence Erlbaum, Hillsdale, N.J., 1985, with permission.)

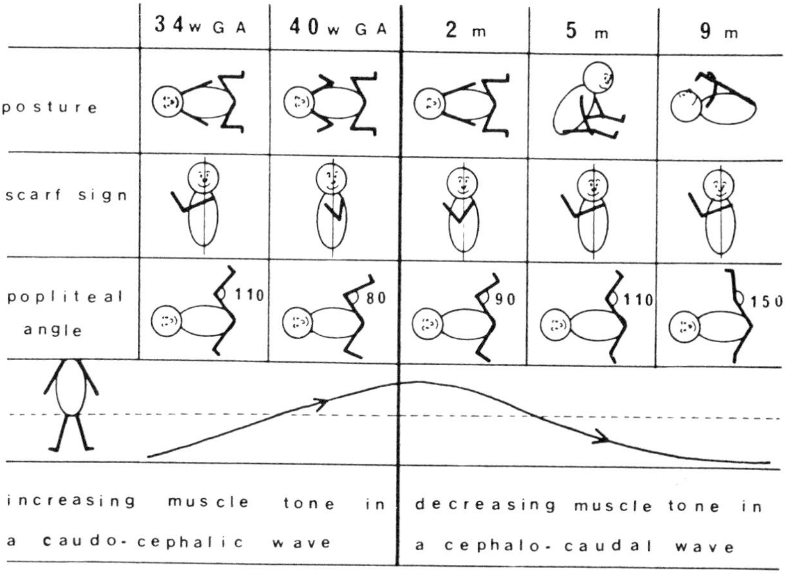

	34 w GA	40 w GA	2 m	5 m	9 m
posture					
scarf sign					
popliteal angle	110	80	90	110	150

increasing   muscle   tone   in   decreasing   muscle   tone   in
a   caudo-cephalic   wave   a   cephalo-caudal   wave

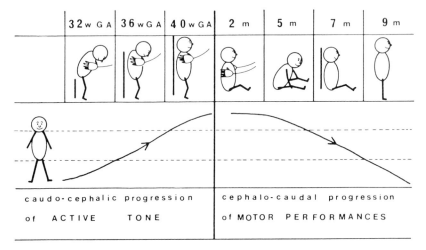

Fig. 3-2 Active tone in the axis. From 28 to 40 weeks GA, when the infant is held in the upright position, a righting reaction first appears in the legs, later in the trunk, and finally in the neck, and is maintained for a few seconds. Within the first year of life, head control is acquired first, later the sitting position; finally, around 9 months, the infant can stand up and maintain the standing position for a while. From about 4 to 7 months, no righting reaction is observed when the infant is held in the upright position, at the time when sitting position is being acquired.
(From Amiel-Tison C. In: *Neonate cognition*, J. Mehler and R. Fox (Eds.). Lawrence Erlbaum, Hillsdale, N.J., 1985, with permission.)

Maturation then slows somewhat, but it is still possible to define monthly or trimestrial stages. Parallel to this, there is the progression of tonic acquisition; from 40 weeks GA this development follows a descending wave of acquisition that is very similar to the ascending wave seen in the third trimester of pregnancy. That is for passive tone, flexor tone of the extremities will decrease starting with the upper extremities proceeding to the lower extremities to result in physiological hypotonia typically seen at 8 months (Fig. 3-1). There is great individual variation in the degree of maximum hypotonia and the pattern in which it is attained, but the cephalocaudal direction is a constant phenomenon that allows the demonstration of anomalies.

Acquisition in the cephalocaudal direction also occurs for active tone (Fig. 3-2). Head control is acquired first, then the ability to sit, and finally the ability to stand.

Description of Techniques

PHYSICAL EXAMINATION OF THE SKULL

Head circumference

Head circumference should be measured at each visit and recorded on the head circumference growth curve. By comparing the slope of the infant's head growth curve with that of the normal curve, it is possible (even during the first months of life) to determine whether head growth approaches the normal range or whether the infant is at risk for development of either hydrocephalus or microcephaly. We use the curves of Nelhaus [7], with corrected age (Fig. 3-3). Head circumference growth is a major piece of data in the first trimester whether the infant was born at term or prematurely.

Anterior fontanelle and sutures

Because of the variability in normal size, we indicate on the grid only whether the fontanelle is tense or depressed. The fontanelle should be palpated while the infant is in a sitting position and not crying. The normal range for the separation of sutures is a function of both the infant's age and the suture being examined. For the sagittal and parieto-occipital sutures, separations of as much as 4 or 5 mm may be of no significance during the first weeks of life. Separations of 4 or 5 mm can also be observed without significance in the portion of the metopic and coronal sutures close to the angles of the anterior fontanelle.

However, separation of 2 to 3 mm of the *squamous suture* (parieto-temporal) is alarming and can be a reliable sign of ICH. If this is suspected, the skull must be reexamined every 2–3 days in order to monitor the tension of the fontanelles, any progressive enlargement of all sutures, or a rapid increase in head size. Additional procedures should be included in the workup if there is a suspicion of hydrocephalus or ICH. Only rarely will a single measurement be of any significance; however, repeated measurements and evaluation of the growth curve will be useful in making a diagnosis.

By contrast, rapid closure of the anterior fontanelle and the squamous suture, with ossification and overriding of the temporal bone on the parietal (edge palpable) and disturbing signs suggesting cerebral atrophy.

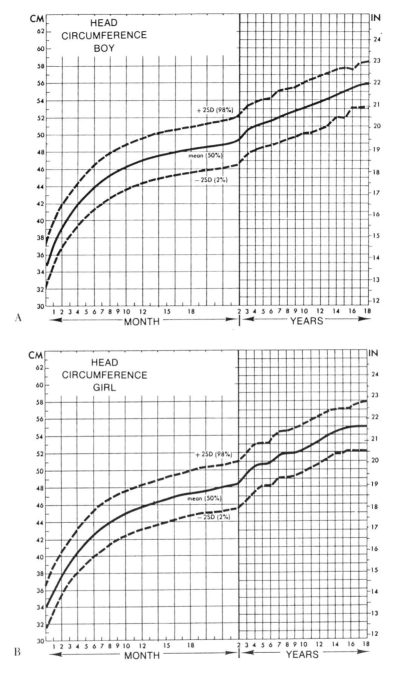

Fig. 3-3 Head circumference charts. (A) Males, (B) Females.
(From Nelhaus G. Composite international and interracial graphs. *Pediatrics,*
41, 106, 1968, with permission.)

HISTORICAL INFORMATION COLLECTED
FROM THE MOTHER

An interview with the mother or nurse is extremely important and can contribute more relevant information than may be obtained from a number of sophisticated procedures. Without this interview, the examination would be incomplete.

Sleep patterns

The mother or nurse should be asked to make a rough estimation of the infant's usual patterns for wakefulness and sleep. Interpretation of the response is dependent on the infant's age and on the absence of nutritional problems. Three abnormal situations can be identified, each specific to a different age and developmental state:

1. The infant sleeps for only very brief periods during the day, is agitated, and cries as soon as awake. The infant is never in a quiet, alert state; rather, the infant appears to be in a permanent state of agitation and discomfort. This pattern is observed most commonly during the first months of life.
2. The infant is quiet during the day but has great difficulty falling asleep at night. Sleep is preceded by a prolonged period of drowsiness. This pattern is more often noted in the third or fourth trimesters.
3. The infant sleeps for excessively long periods—far too long for a 24-hour period. The infant is constantly drowsy. It is difficult, if not impossible, to arouse the infant completely, and the infant will remain awake for only very brief periods.

The infant's arousal state during the tests should be noted on the form, even though this represents only an imprecise estimation of alertness. The examination should be repeated if the infant is unusually agitated, as reported by the mother, or if the behavior interferes with testing. If assessments were carried out under difficult conditions, this should be noted on the examination form.

Quality of cry

The cry should be described as normal or abnormal. An abnormal cry is either high-pitched, monotonous, moaning, continuous, or weak, or a cry that is accompanied by cyanosis or vasomotor instability.

Sucking behavior

Sucking and swallowing coordination should be evaluated and recorded as either normal or abnormal. It should be noted if gavage feeding is necessary or if only partial bottle-feeding is possible. Frequent choking during feeding—either with or without cyanosis—should be noted on the grid.

Convulsions during the preceding months

Convulsions may be generalized or localized, febrile or nonfebrile, infantile spasms, or salaam seizures (hypsarrhythmia).

ABNORMAL OCULAR SIGNS

Hypertonia of elevators palpebrae superiori

In infants with hypertonia of the upper eyelids, the upper part of the sclera and entire iris are visible; however, the globe of the eye is positioned normally. This is in contrast to the sunset sign, in which the globe is lowered abnormally into the orbit. It is essential to distinguish these two conditions; one is not a mild form of the other. Generally, hypertonia of the elevator muscles of the upper eyelids is not an isolated finding and is observed in the context of a general hyperexcitability.

Sunset sign

The sunset sign results from a downward rotation of the ocular globes. As a result, the lower eyelids partially cover the iris, and the sclera above the iris is visible. The sign may be present at all times or in some cases may be elicited during the examination.

Marked strabismus

Marked strabismus may be either convergent or divergent, unilateral or bilateral. A constant ocular deviation after age 5 months requires an examination by a specialist.

Sustained nystagmus

Pendular nystagmus might be indicative of a visual deficit of either central or peripheral origin. The ocular globes do not remain directed toward an object and are constantly animated in a sustained pendular movement. It is a sensorial deficit that prevents fixation on an object. Specialized examinations are clearly essential.

SENSORY DEVELOPMENT

Evaluation of visual and auditory function is included in cognitive developmental assessments. However, two simple maneuvers can be carried out as part of the neurological examination during the neonatal period. Once an appropriate response has been documented, the maneuvers need not be repeated.

Visual pursuit

The infant must be in a quiet, alert state. The synergy between sucking and opening of the eyes can facilitate this observation. During the neonatal period, it is possible to evaluate visual pursuit by using a light source, an object, or the face of the observer. The light source can be either a small flashlight or a window emitting a moderately bright light. The infant will direct his head toward the light source, and, if the body is turned to either side, the eyes will remain fixed on the light. Earlier the use of a glossy "bull's-eye" of concentric black and white circles was mentioned (see Chapter 2).

Acoustic blink reflex

This reflex is elicited by a hand clap at a distance of ~30 cm from the infant's ear. The infant will respond positively to this stimulus by blinking.

POSTURE AND SPONTANEOUS MOTOR ACTIVITY

We preface our discussion by reminding the reader that certain postures or movements might be present consistently, whereas others will be exhibited only occasionally, or will indicate the positions preferred by the infant. Because various prognostic importance has been attached to certain characteristics of these movements, it is essential to observe the infant carefully before assigning a diagnosis or interpreting the results.

Asymmetric tonic neck reflex (spontaneous or postural)

This reflex is observed in an infant lying in the supine position with the head turned to one side. The *fencing position* is exhibited in the

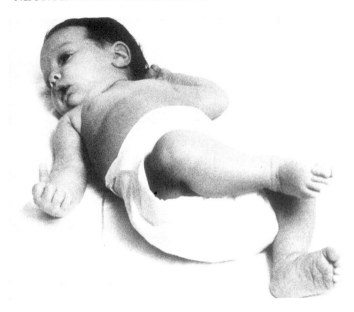

Fig. 3-4 Asymmetric tonic neck reflex (postural). "Fencing position" is observed.

extension of the arm on the side toward which the face is turned; the occipital arm remains flexed. The position is reversed in the lower extremities (i.e., occipital leg extended, opposite leg flexed) (Fig. 3-4).

Although the asymmetric tonic neck reflex can involve both the upper and lower extremities, it is considered to be present if noted in the posture of either the arms or the legs. The reflex is observed during the first 3 months of life and can be noted intermittently from the third to sixth month. It is not present in the normal child after 6 months of age.

Abnormal hypertonia of neck extensors

When the infant rests in a supine position, the neck is normally flexed, the muscles are relaxed, and there is little or no space between the cervical spine and the examination table. This is true throughout all developmental phases (Fig. 3-5A).

When there is a hypertonicity of the neck extensors, an infant placed in the supine position cannot lie completely flat, thereby leaving a space between the neck and the examination table (Fig. 3-5B). As a conse-

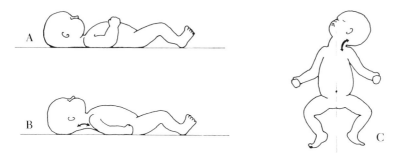

Fig. 3-5 Abnormal hypertonia of extensor muscles of neck. (A) Normal posture, minimal free space; (B) some free space between neck and examination table. (C) Resting posture in lateral rotation, with posterior extension of head in relationship to axis of trunk.

quence, the infant's resting posture will assume a lateral decubitus position with posterior extension of the head (Fig. 3-5C).

Note: The typically deformed head and prominent occiput of a former premature infant can complicate interpretation of this sign. In such instances, interpretation must be consistent with other signs testing the same muscle groups, such as repeated ventral flexion of the head (see below).

Opisthotonos

A permanent hypertonicity of the extensor muscles of the spine maintains the back in an arched position. The infant cannot lie flat in the supine position and will assume a lateral decubitus position with hyperextension when resting.

Permanent closure of the hands

Although the newborn's hands generally remain closed, the hands open and close frequently while resting quietly. The hands are open most of the time after 2 months of age (Fig. 3-6). Special note should be made if the thumb is adducted and flexed across the palm in the clenched fist.

Asymmetric posture of limbs

In order to determine symmetry in the posture of the upper extremities, the head must be aligned carefully with the axis of the trunk. Permanent asymmetry in posture would indicate asymmetry in the

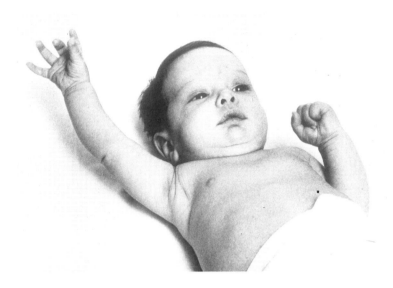

Fig. 3-6   Spontaneous opening and closing of hands in 2-month-old infant.

passive tone. This abnormality would be confirmed by specific maneuvers described later in this examination.

Facial paralysis

Paralysis is most apparent when the infant is crying. The affected side remains flaccid or masklike, and the mouth is drawn toward the opposite side. The eye of the affected side remains partially open, whereas the eyelids close on the normal half of the face.

Spontaneous motor activity

NORMAL MOVEMENTS.   The infant is observed while lying supine on the examination table. The frequency and intensity of spontaneous movement are noted; however, as the examiner's observations represent no more than a gross estimate of motor activity, only significant deviations from normal are recorded. Decreased spontaneous motor activity is characterized by slow, infrequent movements and low intensity. Excessive spontaneous motor activity is expressed in frequent, rapid movements with a very high level of intensity. Normal motility is represented by a mean range in the frequency, intensity, and speed of movements. Asymmetry is noted if the spontaneous activity of one limb is rare or absent as compared with the other side.

Spontaneous motor activity is normally very variable. Movements that are stereotyped, repeated, and identical are considered abnormal. Examples of such movements are pedaling of the legs and making windmills with the arms.

ABNORMAL MOVEMENTS.   These may appear in a permanent or transient manner.

Continuous Tremors. These can be either transient or permanent. Continuous tremors (high frequency, low amplitude) are not uncommon in full-term infants during the first few days of life. The tremors, which are increased by hunger and crying, are most obvious in the extremities and the maxilla and may be significant if persistent, or if present when the infant is at rest.

Bursts of Clonic Movements. Bursts of clonic movements (low frequency, high amplitude) are associated with the Moro reflex or with the spontaneous motor activity of infants during the first hours of life. If the movements are noted frequently during the examination, they may be significant.

Other Abnormal Movements. Other examples of abnormal motor behavior include incessant chewing movements, frequent jerking, and abnormal positioning of the arms, characterized by an extension of the elbows and pronation of the wrists.

Labile stiffening (dyskinetic movements of the limbs)

Labile stiffening can be observed during examination of the limbs. Although subject to possible criticism, the term "labile" provides an appropriate description of this finding in both active and passive movements. Stiffening may vary in intensity and duration (i.e., 10–20 seconds). The involved muscle groups may change as well. Lower extremities, including the foot, are typically hyperextended. In the upper extremities, pronation of the forearm is commonly observed. These dyskinetic movements can impede assessment of passive tone, particularly in the dorsiflexion of the foot. If pronation is present, the application of slow and rapid movements used in testing dorsiflexion must be carried out between bursts of labile stiffening.

PASSIVE TONE

Evaluation of passive tone is determined by the extensibility and amplitude of flapping in different segments of the extremities.

The infant's level of alertness is an important consideration in these evaluations. It is recognized, however, that optimal levels (i.e., states 3 and 4) will not be present during each examination. A less than ideal situation is acceptable as the examination is proposed for use in routine office visits. Findings should be disregarded only if the infant seems to be particularly drowsy or extremely agitated. In testing extensibility, the examiner must be careful to exert no more than a moderate force. Maneuvers are stopped when the infant shows any sign of discomfort.

We have adhered to classical descriptions of the examination, the goal being to evaluate neurological function rather than to examine the joint. Asymmetry, (i.e., *hemisyndrome* or *segmental asymmetry*) may be noticed during the examination.

Extremities

ADDUCTORS ANGLE.   With the infant lying supine, the legs are extended and gently pulled as far apart as possible (Fig. 3-7). The angle formed by the legs at this point is called the adductors angle. Asymmetry between the right and left leg should be noted.

HEEL–EAR MANEUVER.   With the infant lying supine, the legs are held together and pressed as far as possible toward the ears (Fig. 3-8A,B). The pelvis must not be lifted from the table. The angle is represented by the arc extending from the infant's heel to the table. In-

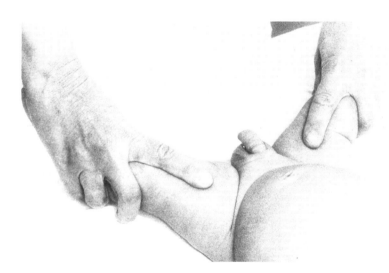

Fig. 3-7 Evaluation of adductors angle. Visualization of angle is simplified by placing index finger on femoral diaphysis.

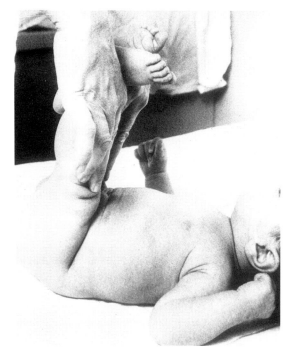

A

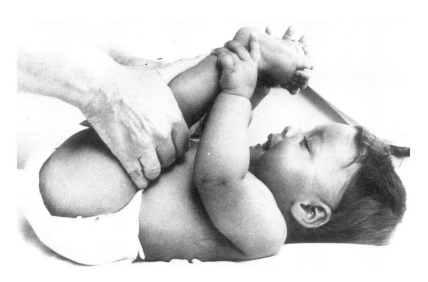

B

Fig. 3-8 Evaluation of heel–ear angle. (A) 100-degree angle in 2-month-old infant. (B) 150-degree angle in 9-month-old infant.

creased resistance on one side is an indication of asymmetry, but it might be difficult to apply equal pressure to both sides.

Note: if there is excessive flexor tone, complete extension of the popliteal angle might be difficult or impossible to accomplish. In this event, the angle is not that formed by the thigh and the table; rather, it is created by an imaginary line between the heel and the pelvis at the intersection with the table.

HYPERFLEXION OF THE HIPS.   If the hips are fixed in a hyperflexed posture, it will be painful or even impossible to extend the lower limbs. Such hyperflexion is considered an abnormal sign if persistent beyond the first weeks of life.

POPLITEAL ANGLE.   The thighs are flexed laterally at the hip along both sides of the abdomen. While holding the infant in this position, the examiner presses the lower leg as far as possible toward the thigh (Fig. 3-9A,B). The popliteal angle, which is formed by the calf and the thigh, is estimated in both legs simultaneously. In contrast to the maneuvers described above, it is easier to apply equal pressure to both sides when examining the popliteal angle; therefore, estimation of asymmetry is more objective. Significant asymmetry is indicated by a difference of 10 to 20 degrees between the right and left angles.

Note: All the preceding maneuvers may be influenced by the fetal position *in utero*. The delivery records should be reviewed if these maneuvers demonstrate extreme hyperextension of the lower extremities persistent over the first few months of life. A breech delivery or breech presentation, even after external or spontaneous rotation, may be significant.

DORSIFLEXION ANGLE OF THE FOOT.   The examiner holds the infant's leg straight and flexes the foot toward the leg. This is accomplished by applying pressure with the thumb to the sole of the foot. The dorsiflexion angle is formed by the dorsum of the foot and the anterior aspect of the leg (Fig. 3-10). This two-phase maneuver is carried out on each side independently. First, a slow, moderate pressure is applied to measure the smallest dorsiflexion angle, called the slow angle. This is followed by a quick, sudden flexion to determine the "rapid" angle. Normally, both angles are equal. A difference between the rapid and slow angles of >10 degrees indicates an abnormally exaggerated stretch reflex.

Response to stretch: phasic contraction and tonic contraction. A rapid dorsiflexion movement can elicit two types of response. These can be distinguished clinically or by electromyography.

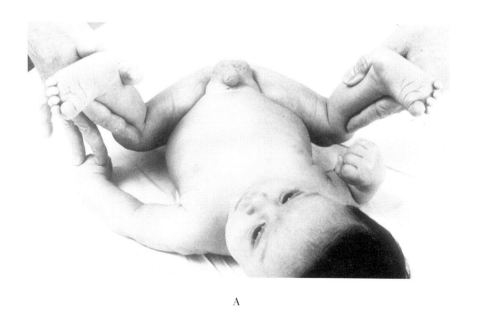

A

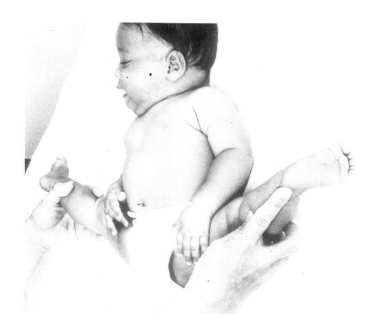

B

Fig. 3-9   Evaluation of popliteal angle. (A) 100-degree angle in 2-month-old infant. (B) 160-degree angle in 9-month-old infant.

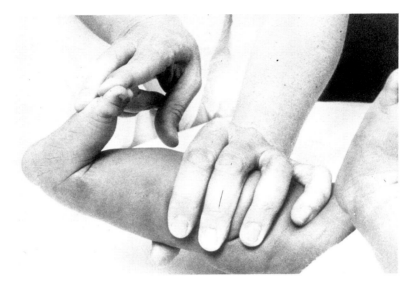

Fig. 3-10 Evaluation of dorsiflexion angle of foot. Flexion of foot with leg held in extension; 50-degree angle in 2-month-old infant.

- A brief contraction immediately followed by a relaxation is called a phasic contraction.
- Sustained resistance to rapid movements followed by slow relaxation thereby returning to the "slow angle" is called a tonic contraction.

Note: Gestational age is significant in the expression of this angle during the neonatal period and the first few months of life. Among premature infants, an angle of <60 degrees would be unusual during the first year of life. This angle is measured with the knee extended in order to evaluate the whole triceps. Only the soleus muscle is tested with the knee in flexion, as the gastrocnemius muscles are excluded by flexion of the knee.

SCARF SIGN. The infant is held in a semireclining position supported by the examiner's palm. At the same time, the examiner takes the infant's hand and pulls the arm as far as possible across the chest toward the opposite shoulder (Fig. 3-11). Three positions are possible in describing the position of the elbow in relationship to the umbilicus:

1. The elbow does not reach midline (score 1).
2. The elbow passes across the midline (score 2).
3. The movement is exaggerated, that is, the arm encircles the neck

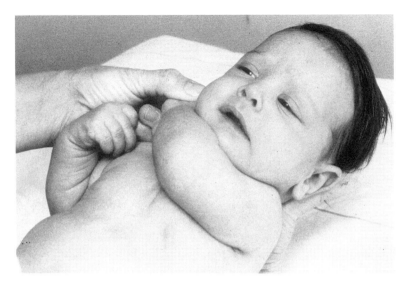

Fig. 3-11 Evaluation of scarf sign. Infant is supported in semireclining position. Elbow reaches midline in 2-month-old infant.

like a scarf, indicating very little resistance in the shoulder muscle (score 3).

Note: The scarf sign may be limited if the infant is obese or extremely irritable during the examination. If either of these conditions is present, this should be noted on the grid.

FLAPPING OF THE FOOT.   Amplitude of movement is assessed by flapping both feet simultaneously at the ankle. The examiner should note any differences in the movement between the right and the left foot (Fig. 3-12).

SQUARE WINDOW.   The hand is flexed as far as possible over the forearm to determine the minimum angle between the palm and the flexor surface of the forearm. In this maneuver, we are interested in asymmetric findings rather than amplitude of the angle (Fig. 3-13).

FLAPPING OF THE HANDS.   Both hands are flapped simultaneously at the wrist. Any significant asymmetry in the amplitude of the movement is noted (Fig. 3-14).

LATERAL ROTATION OF THE HEAD.   The resistance of the contralateral muscles is evaluated by turning the head toward each shoulder (Fig. 3-15). Any significant asymmetry is recorded; however, the am-

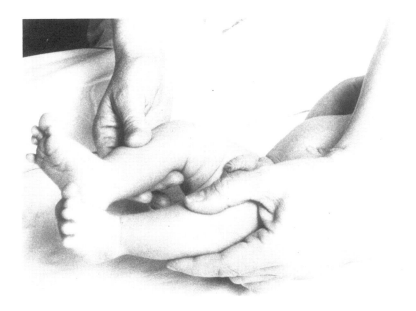

Fig. 3-12   Simultaneous evaluation of flapping of both feet.

Fig. 3-13   Evaluation of square window. Flexion of hands over forearm.

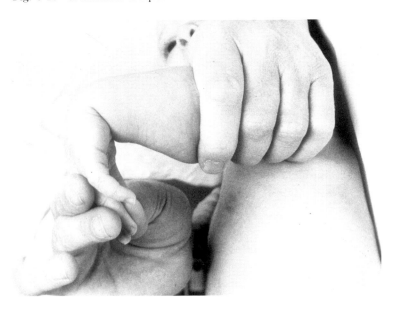

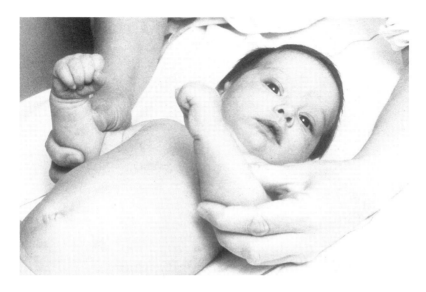

Fig. 3-14   Simultaneous evaluation of flapping in both hands.

Fig. 3-15   Lateral rotation of head.

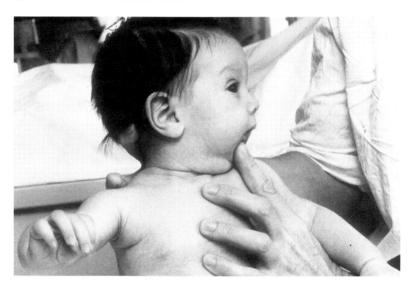

plitude of movement is not interpreted, as it is not important in the absence of asymmetry.

Spinal Axis

REPEATED VENTRAL FLEXION OF THE HEAD.   Repeated flexion of the neck normally causes no changes in the resistance of antagonist muscles. Hypertonicity of the extensors is indicated by increased resistance on repeated flexion (Fig. 3-16). Strongest resistance is reached in most cases after four to five flexions. The head may remain temporarily fixed in hyperextension.

VENTRAL FLEXION OF THE TRUNK.   The legs and hips are pushed toward the head in order to achieve a maximum incurvation of the trunk (Fig. 3-17). Some passive flexion of the trunk is normal; however, this flexion is usually limited and may be impeded further by the volume of the abdomen. If the movement is exaggerated, the knees will touch the chin without difficulty. Flexion may be impossible, in which case the trunk remains rigid and is lifted without flexion.

EXTENSION OF THE TRUNK.   With the infant in lateral decubitus, the examiner holds the lumbar spine with one hand and pulls both legs backward with the other (Fig. 3-18). Extension is normally very limited, if present at all. In an exaggerated response, the dorsal curve is

Fig. 3-16   Repeated ventral flexion of head. Evaluation of resistance after repeated flexion of head.

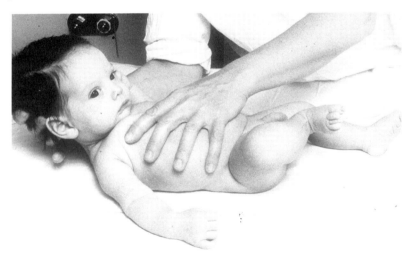

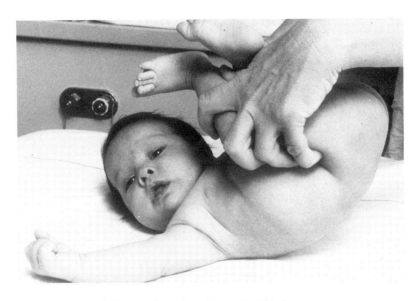

Fig. 3-17   Ventral flexion of trunk in 2-month-old infant.

Fig. 3-18   Absence of incurvation of trunk in dorsal extension maneuver. One hand supports lumbar spine.

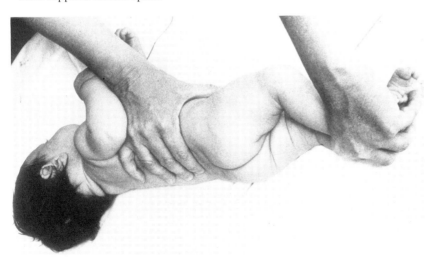

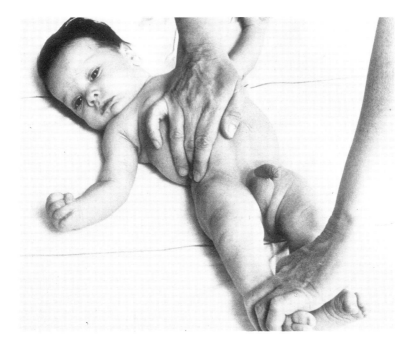

Fig. 3-19 Lateral flexion of trunk. One hand holds flank in position.

less pronounced than the flexion curve. The absence of any extension curvature is not pathological and is considered normal at all ages.

Note: It is difficult to quantitate ventral flexion, especially since ventral flexion increases with age. During the third and fourth trimesters, it is not abnormal for the knees to touch the chin without difficulty. Accordingly, it is more useful to compare the relative values of the extension and flexion curves, rather than to evaluate each curve independently:

• Increased flexion and extension curves are consistent with general hypotonia of the trunk.
• An increased extension curve without flexion may indicate hypertonia of the spinal extensors.

LATERAL FLEXION OF THE TRUNK.   The infant is placed in a supine position. While holding one flank in place, the examiner pulls both legs as far as possible in that direction, thereby producing an incurvation of the trunk. This maneuver is repeated on the opposite side (Fig. 3-19). Movement reflects the tonicity of the contralateral muscles and is normally very limited. Either pronounced incurvation or asymmetry would be an important finding.

ACTIVE TONE

A significant part of the grid is used in the evaluation of active tone. This is not the same as the complementary neuromotor examination described below, since the responses tested here are simple segmented responses that can be coded and compared.

We refer to the neck muscles in describing the technique used to study active segmental reaction. In this example, coordinated reaction of the neck muscles is stimulated by the examiner's movement of the trunk. The appropriate speed for this maneuver must be acquired by experience: if it is done too briskly, passive mobilization of the head may result; if too slowly, the lack of active response may be interpreted incorrectly as abnormal.

When the examination is carried out correctly, abnormal response at any age is alarming. Because of the subjectivity inherent in this evaluation, the examiner's experience is of great importance. Accordingly, conclusions should be made on the basis of repeated assessment. Integrity of motor function and the transient nature of any segmental anomaly will be confirmed by normal response to the lateral abduction reaction, as described later. If initial maneuvers reveal normal segmental response, further examinations will not be necessary.

"Raise to sit" maneuver: evaluation of neck flexors

The infant lying supine is grasped by the shoulders and raised into a sitting posture. Movement from the supine position should be neither too brisk nor too slow. This maneuver elicits reaction of the neck flexors, as observed in the position of the head. Active contractions of neck flexors bring the head forward before the trunk reaches a full vertical position (Fig. 3-20A). Flexor and extensor tone are normally balanced in the full-term infant, resulting in a momentary alignment of the head and trunk (Fig. 3-20B) prior to a forward drop of the head onto the chest (Fig. 3-20C). The following are considered abnormal responses to this maneuver.

- Forward flexion of the head is *difficult* to obtain, maintain, or repeat.
- The response is *absent;* that is, the head remains passive when aligned with the axis of the trunk and falls forward immediately when brought into the full vertical position (i.e., passive forward movement).

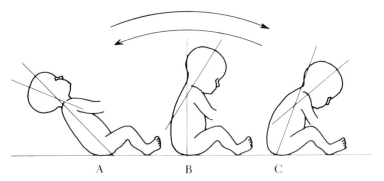

Fig. 3-20   Raise-to-sit maneuver and return backward. Normal response in a full-term newborn; the head actively follows the movement of the trunk from back to front (A–C) and then from front to back (C–A) with well-controlled movement of the head in the axis.

- The response is *impossible*. The head is far back from the beginning of the movement (Fig. 3-21A), does not pass in the axis when the trunk is vertical (Fig. 3-21B), and will not fall forward at the end of this maneuver (Fig. 3-21C). The position of the chin (projected forward) and the impossibility of active forward motion of the head is the easiest abnormal pattern to identify. These findings indicate either a hypertonicity of the extensors of the neck or a hypotonicity of the flexors.

Fig. 3-21   Raise-to-sit maneuver and return backward. Abnormal response by imbalance of tone favoring the extensor muscles of the neck, resulting (A, B) in inability of the head to move forward and (C) inability of the head to fall forward on the chest.

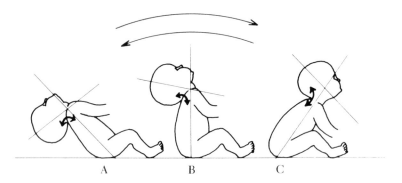

Lowering from sitting to supine position: evaluation of neck extensors

The maneuver begins with the infant in a sitting position and the head dropped forward onto the chest (Fig. 3-20C). The infant is grasped by the shoulders and moved backward. Movement must be neither too brisk nor too slow. Mobilization of the trunk should elicit contraction of the neck extensors, resulting in an active lifting of the head (Fig. 3-20B,A). This reaction should be noted carefully by the examiner. In the normal infant, an alternate contraction of the neck extensors and flexors is elicited by a gentle rocking motion at the vertical axis with the trunk. This is described as *symmetrical braking* and is normal in the full-term infant during the first days of life. The following are considered abnormal responses:

- Head movement is *difficult* to elicit, cannot be obtained repeatedly, or is described as brisk and unbalanced.
- The response is *absent*. The head is flexed forward on the chest at the onset of the maneuver, passes passively through the vertical axis,, and falls backward with all of its weight.
- The response is *"too good."* There is a permanent imbalance of the flexors and extensors of the neck that favors the extensors: at the beginning of the maneuver the head is not lying forward on the chest (Fig. 3-21C). As soon as the trunk is moved backward the head moves immediately backward (Fig. 3-21B,A). Symmetrical braking of the head does not exist in this case.

The frequently encountered difficulty in interpreting these two maneuvers comes from the impossibility of testing the flexors and extensors individually, as they are antagonists. However, the combination of the impossibility of active forward motion of the head and the response to backward motion that is "too good" affirms the predominance of the extensors of the neck over the flexors. This predominance is most likely a result of a permanent hypertonicity of the neck extensors (frequently accompanied by an abnormal posture of permanent opisthotonos).

Conversely, when there is the isolated finding of a response backward that is "too good" (but the head can drop forward normally), this most likely indicates a weakness of the flexors of the neck (frequently associated with an exaggerated response to the scarf maneuver).

Head control

During the first several months of life, an infant placed in a sitting position cannot align the head with the axis of the trunk for more than

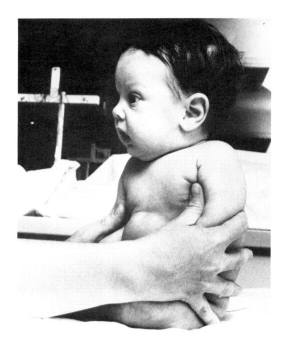

Fig. 3-22 Excellent head control in sitting position in 2-month-old infant.

a few seconds. The head wavers to the side or drops forward. Head control improves with age, and between the second and fourth months the infant should be able to maintain head alignment for ≥15 seconds (Fig. 3-22).

Head control may be impossible, the result of either permanent hypertonicity of neck extensors or significant hypotonia of the neck flexors. Total lack of control is the most severe sign linked with global hypotonia.

Pull-to-sitting position

While lying supine, the infant is encouraged to grasp the examiner's thumbs. Normally, the infant will attempt to pull himself into a sitting position. The examiner follows the infant's movement but provides no special assistance in attempts to achieve this posture (Fig. 3-23).

Note: The infant's voluntary attempt to achieve a sitting position differs considerably from the grasp and traction responses, which represent a generalized tonic flexion of all flexor muscles in the arm and forearm.

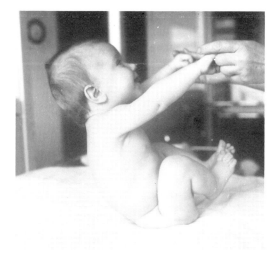

Fig. 3-23 Pull-to-sitting position. A 5-month-old infant pulls on examiner's index fingers to achieve sitting position.

Sitting alone, supported by arms

The infant is placed in a sitting position with hips adducted at ~90 degrees and lower extremities in extension. The body is inclined slightly forward, leaning on the arms. It should be possible for the infant to maintain this position for several seconds (Fig. 3-24). Two types of abnormal positions can be observed:

1. The infant may fall forward between his legs; the trunk remains completely hypotonic and no active attempt to maintain vertical position is noticed (Fig. 3-25).
2. The infant might fall backward because of insufficient tone in the anterior muscle groups or excessive tone in the posterior muscle groups. (Fig. 3-26).

It can be difficult or impossible to place the infant in a sitting position because of decreased extensibility and abnormally strong flexor tone in the lower extremities. The knees may be too high because of a decreased popliteal angle, or the knees may be too close together as the result of a decreased adductor angle (Fig. 3-26). Such decreases in either angle prevent the triangulation in the lower extremities necessary to ensure a good base of support for the sitting posture.

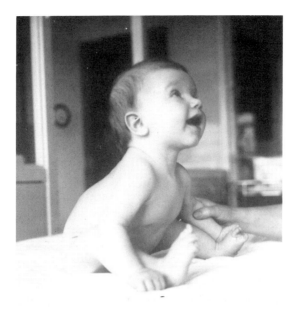

Fig. 3-24 A 5-month-old infant sitting alone for several seconds, using arms for support. Note large support base provided by abduction and extension of lower extremities. Position shown is appropriate for the age.

Sitting alone for ≥30 seconds

The infant is positioned as previously described and is able to sit for at least 30 seconds without support (Fig. 3-27).

Global straightening of the trunk and lower extremities

The infant is maintained in a standing position, supported by the examiner's hand around the chest. The middle finger holds the infant at the axilla and the index finger lifts the chin. By straightening the lower

Fig. 3-25 Sitting position is impossible, the hypotonic trunk falling *forward* between the legs.

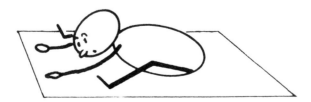

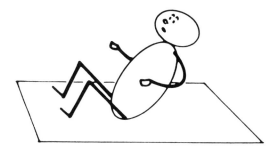

Fig. 3-26 Sitting position is impossible. Knees are high and close together; infant falls *backward*.

Fig. 3-27 Sitting alone without support. Appropriate sitting position in 9-month-old infant.

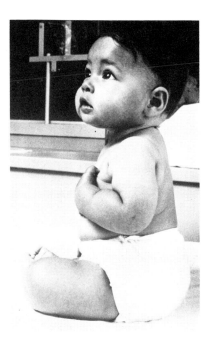

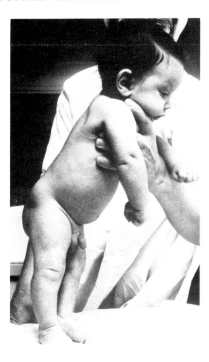

Fig. 3-28   Straightening with lower limbs and trunk in a 2-month-old infant.

extremities—that is, contracting the spinal muscles—the infant should be able to support himself in this position for several seconds without additional assistance (Fig. 3-28).

During the first months of life, this straightening reaction is considered present even if the knees remain semiflexed as a result of hypertonicity of the flexor muscles. The reaction disappears over the following several months. During this time, it is impossible for the infant to stand, either by reflex reaction or by voluntary straightening (Fig. 3-29).

At 7 or 8 months when the infant is held firmly below each arm the normal response is a rapid succession of extension then flexion, as if extension cannot be well maintained. This is the "jumping" stage.

Toward 8 or 9 months the infant can support his or her weight in a standing position (Fig. 3-30).

If there is marked hypertonia of the posterior muscles, each attempt at placing the infant in a sitting position will result in global straightening and opisthotonos. This is noted in the grid as "trunk arching."

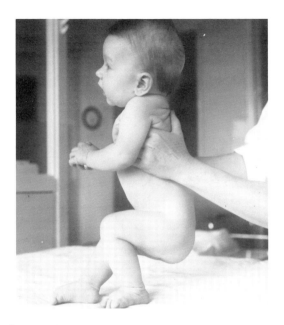

Fig. 3-29 Absence of straightening in a 5-month-old infant. (The same infant is capable of pulling to sitting position actively (Fig. 3-23) and can maintain sitting position without help for a few seconds (Fig. 3-24).

Fig. 3-30 A 9-month-old infant stands alone for an extended period of time.

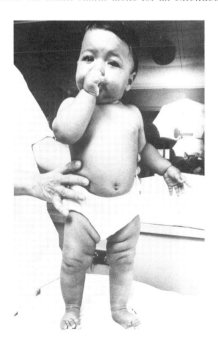

PRIMARY REFLEXES, DEEP TENDON REFLEXES, AND POSTURAL REACTIONS

This section describes some of the primary reflexes present during the first few months of life. While these reflexes may disappear at varying ages, persistence beyond 5 or 6 months is significant. Some deep tendon reflexes are examined routinely. In conclusion, we describe some of the postural reactions that typically appear at a specific age.

Primary Reflexes

AUTOMATIC WALKING.   The infant is supported at the trunk, tilted slightly forward. Automatic walking, produced by contact of the soles of the feet with the solid surface of the examination table, is considered present when the infant takes a few steps (Fig. 3-31).

Automatic walking can persist beyond extinction of the straightening reaction. In this event, the infant's legs will be slightly flexed when walking.

PALMAR GRASP.   The examiner places an index finger in the infant's palm. This palmar stimulation produces flexion of the fingers that decreases with age and disappears between the third and fourth months of life. The maneuver can be carried out on both sides simultaneously (Fig. 3-32A).

RESPONSE TO TRACTION BY THE FLEXORS OF THE UPPER EXTREMITIES.   After eliciting the palmar grasp, the examiner pulls the infant forward, as if lifting the infant—thereby provoking a generalized contraction of flexor muscles in the upper extremities. In this lifting reaction, the infant supports all or a portion of his weight. Tonic response of the flexor muscles is dependent on the *quality of the active tone*.

With excellent active tone, the infant completely lifts his weight in a quite spectacular way; while supporting this weight the infant's head is aligned with the axis of the trunk and the lower extremities are flexed actively for a few seconds (Fig. 3-32B).

At the beginning of the second trimester, the two reflex reactions described above are replaced by active voluntary grasping. The infant will purposely grasp onto the examiner's index finger, pulling on this support to achieve a sitting position. Simultaneous bilateral evaluation of these maneuvers can detect even mild asymmetries

MORO REFLEX.   The supine infant is lifted a few centimeters off the examination table by pulling gently on both hands. Upper extremities are in extension (Fig. 3-33A).

When the hands are released suddenly, the infant falls backward on the examination table and the reflex is manifest (Fig. 3-33B).

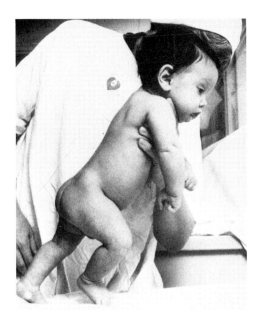

Fig. 3-31 Automatic walking in a 2-month-old infant.

Fig. 3-32 Palmar grasp. (A) Grasping reflex. (B) Response to traction of flexor muscles in upper extremities. This 2-month-old infant is able to support his own weight by grasping onto examiner's index finger.

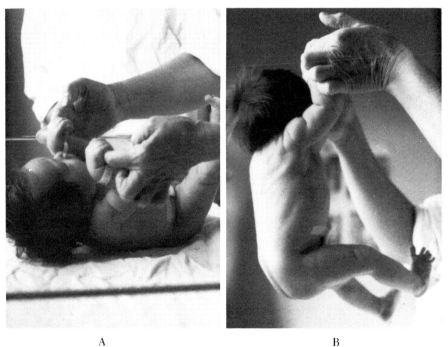

A   B

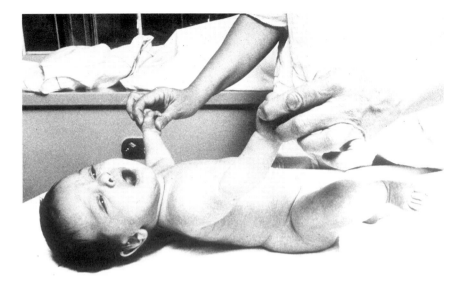

A

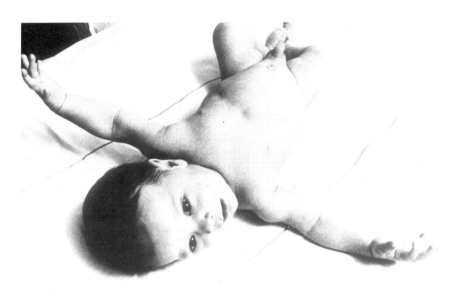

B

Fig. 3-33 Moro reflex, (A) triggered by pulling on both hands, thereby creating space between neck and examination table. (B) First phase of Moro reflex, with abduction and extension of arms. Note flexion of lower limbs, both soles turned inward.

The reflex begins with an abduction of the arms and extension of the forearms. This is followed by adduction and flexion of the forearms. The hands open completely at the onset, and the reflex concludes with the infant crying.

Normal response during the first trimester includes abduction and extension of the forearms, opening of the hands, and, finally, a cry. Adduction and flexion of the forearms may not be present. During the second trimester, the reflex may be incomplete, involving no more than an opening of the hands and a cry. Later, even this incomplete reflex will disappear. At this time, even a minimal response is considered abnormal. The examiner should be alert to the absence of the reflex during the first two trimesters, asymmetric response, or low threshold (i.e., elicitation of the reflex by even slight stimulation). Low threshold is accompanied by a burst of clonic contractions.

EVOKED ASYMMETRIC TONIC NECK REFLEX. With the infant supine, the head is rotated passively in order to change the tone of the extremities. The arm is extended on the side toward which the head is turned. The opposite arm remains in a more flexed position. Only partial response may be noted in the lower extremities, which usually assume a flexion and extension pattern opposite to that seen in the upper extremities. This evoked response is subtle and variable or completely absent in the normal infant. In an abnormal infant, the response is constant, repetitive, stereotyped, and unaffected by spontaneous motor activity.

Deep tendon reflexes

BICEPS REFLEX. With the infant lying supine, the elbow is held in a semiflexed position. The examiner places his or her index finger on the biceps tendon. While maintaining the forearm in semiflexion, the examiner taps the index finger with a reflex hammer or with the index or third finger of the opposite hand. This tapping provokes contraction of the biceps (i.e., flexion of the forearm). Response may be absent, exaggerated, clonic, or diffuse.

KNEE JERK. The infant is placed supine on the examination table and the knee is held in a semiflexed position. The reflex is elicited by tapping the patellar tendon with a reflex hammer, or with the index or third finger. Normally, a sharp tap is followed by contraction of the muscle. The reflex can be absent, exaggerated, clonic, or diffused.

ANKLE CLONUS. The maneuver should be carried out subsequent to relaxation of the leg muscles, with the infant resting quietly in a supine position. A brisk but gentle dorsiflexion of the ankle is achieved

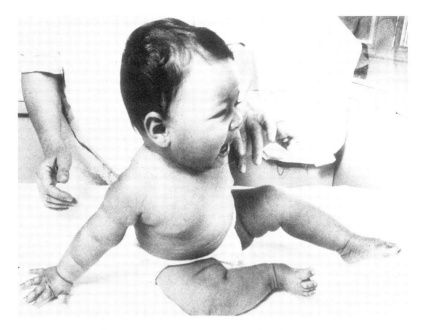

Fig. 3-34 Lateral propping reaction. A 9-month-old infant, sitting alone, extends one arm to prevent falling when pushed laterally by examiner.

with the hip and knee flexed. Ankle clonus is manifest in a rhythmic series of alternating contractions and partial relaxations of the foot at the ankle. A few rapidly fading contractions are normal in the newborn; however, clonus persisting beyond 10 contractions is considered abnormal.

Vestibular and visual postural reactions

We will not debate the issue of whether the primary stimulus is vestibular or visual; however, it is apparent that the lateral propping reaction and parachute reaction are hallmarks of normal development. Both are of great interest clinically.

LATERAL PROPPING REACTION. This reaction usually appears between 6 and 8 months, after the baby is able to sit alone without assistance. The examiner pushes the baby to one side with a sudden shove of the shoulder. In response, the baby should extend the appropriate arm to prevent falling. Absence of the reaction or asymmetric response should be noted (Fig. 3-34).

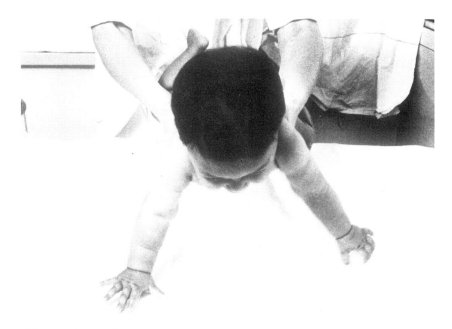

Fig. 3-35 Parachute maneuver. This 9-month-old infant is thrust forward abruptly toward the examination table. The infant responds with a protective gesture, extending arms and opening hands.

PARACHUTE REACTION.   The baby is held in ventral suspension close to the examiner, then thrust suddenly head-first toward the examination table. In a normal defensive reaction, the baby extends the arms and opens the hands to break the fall (Fig. 3-35). This reflex appears between 7 and 9 months; however, the reaction is delayed in infants with motor difficulty of CNS origin. Absent or asymmetric response should be recorded.

Asymmetric findings in the two maneuvers described above are important in the diagnosis of subtle hemiplegia.

Interpretation of Results

The techniques or the significance of each element of the proposed examination is open to criticism. Some of the criticism is examined below.

EXTENSIBILITY OF THE EXTREMITIES

Individual variation

Considerable individual variation has been shown to exist in the evolution of passive tone during the first year [4,6]; therefore, the range of normal responses is quite large.

The frequent occurrence of benign familial hypotonia is well known. In these cases the evaluation of passive tone can only be made secondarily at the end of the first year. At that time the evolution over the year can be reexamined; it is only in this context that a given extensibility at a given age would have significance as pathological or normal.

Two case histories demonstrate the difficulties of interpretation that are encountered.

> *Case 1.* Elsa B. was born at term following a normal pregnancy, by a difficult midforceps delivery, weighing 4050 g. During the first week of life she had a cluster of neurological signs—specifically an abnormal cry, episodes of cyanosis, hypertonia of the extensors of the neck, and global hypotonia. At the end of the first week, except for persistent global hypotonia, all the signs disappeared. Her subsequent development was normal with the global hypotonia persisting. She did not gain head control until 4 months. At 6 months passive tone was still outside the limits of normal with an adductor angle of 160 degrees, the heel–ear angle at 140 degrees, the popliteal angle at 180 degrees, exaggerated ventral flexion and dorsal extension of the trunk, and an unlimited scarf sign. Questioning of the mother revealed that a maternal uncle, at the time aged 60 years, was still able to place his feet behind his head, an interesting social talent.

Although the monthly evaluations of extensibility were in the abnormal zones, there was in fact normal evolution with benign global hypotonia. Any organic etiology of perinatal origin can be eliminated in this case, and the prognosis is evidently excellent. The minor perinatal signs linked to delivery have no connection with the subsequently observed signs.

> *Case 2.* David P. was a second twin born at 38 weeks GA. He was delivered by breech presentation with no difficulty; he weighed 2470 g, length 44 cm, and head circumference 35.5 cm. The Apgar score was 8 at 1 minute and 10 at 5 minutes, but from birth the baby showed signs of a right subdural hematoma with a bulging and asymmetric fontanelle, disjointive sutures, right retinal hemorrhages that appeared to be old, and permanent opisthotonos. However, he had a normal state of consciousness, good sucking, and normal reflexes. A right subdural puncture produced 35 ml of dark serosanguinous liquid under pressure. On ques-

tioning the mother it was learned that 2 weeks prior to delivery she had fallen on a stairway, landing on her abdomen. It was therefore determined that the subdural hematoma was traumatic in nature. In the days following birth he had no signs of reaccumulation of liquid in the subdural space, and the general evolution was without complication.

However, he had several persistent neurological anomalies. At the age of 7 months, although passive tone was within the limits of normal, there was persistent stiffness of the lower extremities, exaggerated spontaneous motility, moderate to poor active tone of the trunk, and a tendency toward opisthotonos in the examination of passive tone of the trunk. At 8 months his postural ability was still only moderate, with a sitting position like that of a 5-month-old. By contrast, at 10 months the postural acquisitions were within the limits of normal for his age, with good sitting and standing positions and the acquisition of postural reactions.

The motor anomalies were therefore transient, with an abrupt normalization between 8 and 10 months.

If the elements of the evolution of passive tone are examined for this infant, there are two noteworthy facts:

- The evolution toward relaxation of the lower extremities was not smooth; there was an abrupt relaxation between 8 and 10 months (Table 3-1).
- It was possible to use the other twin as a control, since she was perfectly normal at birth.

Until 8 months the extensibility of the control twin was definitely greater, near the upper limits of normal for her age. But at 10 months the extensibility of the two babies was identical; the pathological twin abruptly returned to normal.

Therefore, the evolution of this infant for the first 8 months cannot be considered normal; although extensibility during this time was within the limits of normal, delayed relaxation with abrupt correction at 10 months was observed. The relative hypertonia ended at the typical time when transient problems of tone usually resolve.

Table 3-1 Change in Patterns of Passive Tone in the Lower Extremities—Case 2: David P., Ages 4–8 Months and Abrupt Return to Normal Patterns at 10 Months[a]

	1	2	3	4	5	6	7	8	9	10	11	12
Adductors angle				100	100		110	130		150		
Heel–ear angle				100	100		110	110		140		
Popliteal angle				100	100		110	120		170		

[a] Age in months is indicated at the bottom of each column.

Although after 10 months no difference existed between the baby described and his twin sister who was normal, it is necessary to follow this child until school age. The evolution of these transient motor anomalies during the first year puts him at greater risk for later handicap from the traumatic subdural hematoma that occurred *in utero.*

These two cases demonstrate the necessity of repeated examinations prior to interpretation of results and also show the danger of analysis of raw data. If conclusions were drawn based only on the data, the first case would appear to be that of an infant with abnormality and the second that of a normal infant, when in fact the first case is in the area of benign familial hypotonia and the second is that of lesions of prenatal origin that resulted in transient tonic symptomatology.

Delay in detection of asymmetry of tone of extremities

Recent correlations between clinical and echographic data have confirmed the earlier findings of the clinical delay in diagnosing "congenital hemiplegia," which usually results in clinical signs at ~3 months of age. It is clear that physiological hyperflexion of the extremities renders impossible the detection of asymmetry based on posture or extensibility, that is, up to age 3 months in the upper extremities and to 6 months for the lower extremities. A flexed and inactive thumb, a more brisk return to flexion of the forearm, or an asymmetric posture of the forearms in flexion sometimes brings attention to one side as compared to the other; but it is in these situations that complementary clinical research in the area of active tone is important. For example, in a former premature infant at 3 months corrected age, moderate cerebral atrophy resulted in a left ventricular dilatation *ex vacuo* seen on ultrasound in the sagittal (Fig. 3-36A,B) and median transverse sections (Fig. 3-37), but this was not accompanied by any clinical difference in passive tone on the right side. However the maneuver of lateral support of the arm (see Chapter 4) showed a clear and reproducible deficit in the active performance of the right arm and hand as compared to the left. This moderate deficit was confirmed in follow-up visits observing the child's gross motor control of that hand.

Moderate to poor reproducibility of certain maneuvers

An attempt to measure the interobserver reliability was done in two ways, according to the individuals and their acquired experience [1].

First, two different observers successively examined the same infant without the other present. The results were excellent for the scarf sign and the angle of dorsiflexion of the foot at ±10 degrees, acceptable for the popliteal angle, and poor for the heel–ear maneuver and the ad-

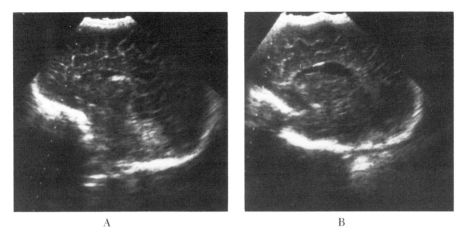

A   B

Fig. 3-36 Echography in right (A) and left (B) sagittal section in a case of moderate cerebral atrophy showing left ventricular dilatation.

ductors angle (Figs. 3-38 and 3-39A). The second test of reliability was performed by only one person and evaluated simultaneously by five observers; the maneuver chosen was the adductors angle. The results were very satisfying with a margin of difference at ±10 degrees (Fig. 3-39B). This demonstrates that the difficulty is not in the visualization of the angle but in the experience and patience of the examiner in performing the maneuver itself. Therefore, any instrument for measuring angles is of no great value; it is more important for the examiner

Fig. 3-37 Echography in transverse median section in the same case of moderate cerebral atrophy as in Fig. 3-36.

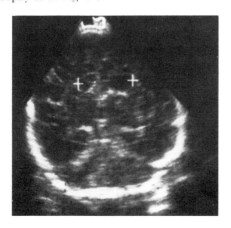

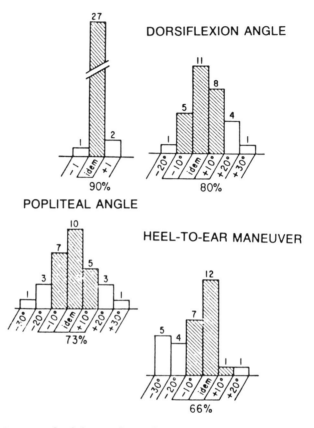

Fig. 3-38 Reproducibility in the evaluation of passive tone. Results obtained by several examiners evaluating the scarf sign, the angle of dorsiflexion of the foot, the popliteal angle, and the heel–ear maneuver in 30 infants.

to gain experience. This also shows that whenever possible it is preferable for an infant to be followed by the same examiner during the first years.

SOME CHARACTERISTICS OF AXIAL TONE

Hypotonia of the flexors of the neck and trunk

When there are abnormalities of axial tone, the anterior muscles, or flexors, are the first and most strongly affected as compared with the

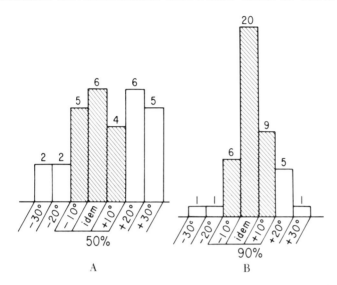

Fig. 3-39   Reproducibility in the evaluation of passive tone. (A) The adductors angle with the maneuver being done by several examiners successively. (B) The adductors angle with the maneuver being done by one examiner with the result evaluated simultaneously by several observers.

posterior or extensor muscles; an imbalance arises with predominance of the extensors. This is explained by the recent observations that the subcortical pathways, responsible for extension, mature earlier and are less vulnerable to hypoxia than the corticospinal tract, which is responsible for flexion of the neck and trunk [8]. If there is a major anomaly there is significant and permanent opisthotonos; when placed in a sitting position the infant straightens, pushes on his feet and arches in a circle. This can be seen, for example, in postanoxic cerebral necrosis. Head control in the sitting position is therefore impossible. A moderate anomaly will result in late acquisition of head control. If the anomaly is minor it will be noted only through evaluation of the extensibility of the trunk, that is, abnormal dorsal extension as compared with ventral flexion that is limited by the antagonists. These minor symptoms disappear gradually with development.

Hypertonia of the extensor muscles of the neck and trunk

This is the best sign of increased intracranial pressure in the newborn and young infant. It is the equivalent of stiffness of the neck in an older child or adult, and is demonstrated by abnormal posture and the abnormal response of the two muscle groups of the neck to the maneuver of raise to sitting and return. The head is unable to pass forward on the raise to sitting and will not fall forward on the thorax even if the infant is held leaning forward; it is held back by the hypertonic extensors. It must be noted that this can be a labile sign that can disappear within several hours as a result of a diuretic injection or a lumbar puncture [9].

The difficulty is in making the clinical distinction between the two causes of axial imbalance, since the only way to evaluate a group of muscles clinically is in comparison with its antagonists.

Moreover, these two situations often appear successively. For example, a full-term infant with acute fetal distress may have cerebral edema during the first days, causing ICH, which results in a permanent positioning of the head backward secondary to hypertonia of the extensors. After the first few days, if there is a cellular lesion, the weakening of the flexors will be perceptible, thus maintaining the imbalance of the two muscle groups. The maneuver of raise to sitting remains poor. However, in the case of weakness of the flexors the head is able to fall completely forward in the sitting position and there is no increasing resistance with repeated flexion of the head on the trunk. These clinical nuances may seem debatable, but the electromyogram can show a clearer distinction between the two situations—that is, prolonged hypotonia of the flexors resulting from a lesion versus hypertonia of the extensors that lasts as long as the ICH that causes it.

Finally, this imbalance can become fixed and the muscle fibers of the trapezius will shorten if care is not taken with position and active exercises of the muscles to correct this situation early. Permanent opisthotonos no longer has to be a peripheral sequela of a central problem that is itself often transient (see p. 115).

ABNORMAL SEQUENCE OF MOTOR ACQUISITION

It has been seen that a longitudinal point of view is essential to decrease errors of interpretation linked to individual variations of tone. But the understanding of the results of each examination has significance in itself as it allows the clear demonstration of an *abnormal sequence*. The best example of this discordance between 4 and 7 months is given by the comparison of sitting and standing; in fact it is often the mother who notes at the beginning of the consultation that her 6-month-old cannot sit unassisted but always wants to be held in the standing position. In the examination the sitting position is often impossible,

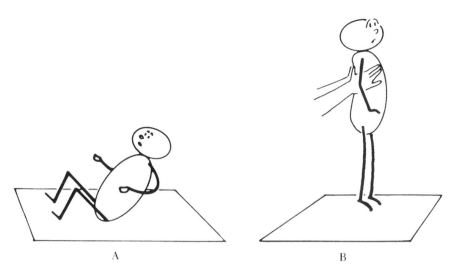

A   B

Fig. 3-40 Discordance between sitting and standing. (A) The baby is unable to sit, falling backward; the knees are raised and close to each other. (B) There is excessive straightening in the standing position on tiptoes, and sometimes a scissor position and a posterior incurvation of the trunk.

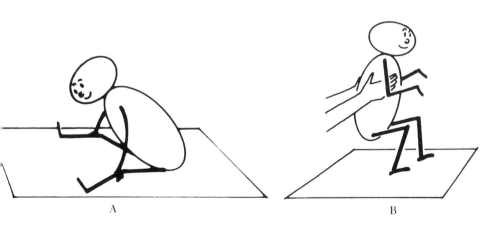

A   B

Fig. 3-41 Normal progression of acquisition in the axis. (A) Sitting unassisted "like at 5 months" with stabilization from the triangle formed by the lower extremities and helped by the arms; the trunk is still leaning forward. (B) Absence of straightening of the lower extremities in the standing position typical of an infant of 5 months (transient absence typical of an infant from 4 to 7 months).

with the baby most often falling backward (Fig. 3-40A), while the standing posture is intense, with marked adduction resulting in a scissor position (Fig. 3-40B). This predominance of extensor tone may not appear on the first attempt but may be encouraged by successive movements of flexion and extension of the lower extremities with plantar contact; there then appears a strong contraction of the extensors.

The normal situation, associated with descending progression of motor acquisition, is just the opposite (see Fig. 3-41A, B).

At the same time, the evaluation of active tone must be carried out in comparison with the evaluation of relaxation of passive tone of the extremities. In fact, the essential prerequisite for sitting is sufficient relaxation of the lower extremities to make a triangular base, with the adductor and popliteal angles almost completely open.

Classification at the End of the First Year

ANALYSIS AND SYNTHESIS

This method of neurological evaluation has not been standardized but is based on data from the literature with regard to the acceptable limits of normal development. As noted above, the main difficulty in the interpretation of results is in the great individual variation of tone. That is the reason it would not be realistic to code the whole grid. This clustering provides the ability to identify several typical profiles of the analytical examination. Clustering of symptoms is a necessary part of the synthesis. Different clusters of symptoms appear more typically at different ages. For this reason a synthesis by trimesters is proposed.

First trimester

During the first trimester, the most frequent moderate anomalies can be separated into two groups: (1) hyperexcitability and (2) a hypotonia of the upper half of the body, with moderate function of the flexors of the head and excessive relaxation of the upper extremities.

In a large majority of cases these signs disappear, often abruptly, in the course of the third month. When seen at 3 months the infant has acquired head control at a normal date, and the hyperexcitability has disappeared. The mother, for whom these two symptoms (agitation and impotence of the neck) are highly noticeable, can often specify the week during which they disappeared. It is not possible to know in advance whether stiffness of the lower extremities will persist, since at this age limited extensibility is normal. It is only by dynamic tests that it is possible to pick up an asymmetry before 3 months of age, which might be the first indication of a spastic hemiplegia.

In the case of extensive cerebral lesions the clinical signs are worrisome immediately: poor contact, difficulty swallowing, little spontaneous motor activity, global hypotonia, and possibly permanent opisthotonos. In these rare cases it is evident from the outset that none of these anomalies will disappear during the first year.

Table 3-2 Most Commonly Observed Transient Neuromotor Anomalies in the First Year of Life

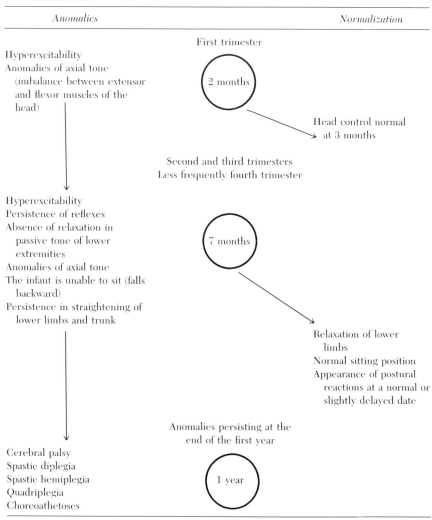

Anomalies		*Normalization*
	First trimester	
Hyperexcitability Anomalies of axial tone (imbalance between extensor and flexor muscles of the head)	2 months	Head control normal at 3 months
	Second and third trimesters Less frequently fourth trimester	
Hyperexcitability Persistence of reflexes Absence of relaxation in passive tone of lower extremities Anomalies of axial tone The infant is unable to sit (falls backward) Persistence in straightening of lower limbs and trunk	7 months	Relaxation of lower limbs Normal sitting position Appearance of postural reactions at a normal or slightly delayed date
	Anomalies persisting at the end of the first year	
Cerebral palsy Spastic diplegia Spastic hemiplegia Quadriplegia Choreoathetoses	1 year	

Second and third trimesters

During the second and third trimesters the most characteristic symptomatology is persistence of hyperexcitability with very active primary reflexes, nonrelaxation of passive tone of the extremities, and imbalance of axial tone with hypotonia of the flexors and relative hypertonia of the extensors of the trunk. On the whole these anomalies can mimic a spastic diplegia, but there are differences. A true spastic diplegia would be indicated by a tight adductors angle with a scissorlike posture, and a strong tonic stretch reflex in the triceps. By contrast, an open adductors angle and a phasic quality of the myotatic reflex indicate that these anomalies are most likely transient. These signs disappear in a dramatic way toward the eighth or ninth month; motor normalization will be complete at 1 year.

In the same way a subtle spastic hemiplegia of perinatal origin, which is usually not diagnosed until around the fifth month of life and is very clear at 6 or 7 months, can totally disappear before the end of the first year.

The most characteristic symptomatic groupings and possible normalization are represented schematically in Table 3-2. The most contributory ages to observe clinically, if a monthly examination is not possible, are 2 months, 7 months, and 1 year corrected age. The three examinations at these ages give the greatest chance of finding transient anomalies. By contrast, only one examination done between 10 months and 1 year will be too late and will not distinguish between the normal infant and one who has normalized at 10 months of age.

References

[1] Amiel-Tison C. A method for neurologic evaluation within the first year of life. In: *Current problems in pediatrics*, VII, no. 1, pp. 1–50. Year Book Medical Publishers, Chicago, 1976.

[2] Amiel-Tison C. A method for neurological evaluation within the first year of life: experience with full-term newborn infants with birth injury. In: *Major mental handicap: methods and costs of prevention*, pp. 107–126. Ciba Foundation Symposium, no. 59, Elsevier, Amsterdam, 1978.

[3] Thomas A. and Ajuriaguerra J. de. *Etude sémiologique du tonus musculaire*. Editions Médicales Flammarion, Paris, 1949.

[4] Stambak M. and Ajuriaguerra J. de. Evolution de l'extensibilité musculaire depuis la naissance jusqu'à 2 ans. *Presse Méd.*, 66, 24–26, 1958.

[5] Touwen B. Neurological development in infancy. *Clinics in developmental medicine*, no. 58, p. 150. Spastic International Medical Publications, London, 1976.

[6] Saint-Anne Dargassies S. *Le développement neuro-moteur et psycho-affectif du nourrisson*, p. 524. Masson, Paris, 1982.

[7] Nelhaus G. Composite international and interracial graphs. *Pediatrics, 41*, 106, 1968.

[8] Sarnat, H. B. Anatomic and physiologic correlates of neurologic development in prematurity. In: *Topics in neonatal neurology*, H. B. Sarnat (Ed.), pp. 1–25. Grune & Stratton, New York, 1984.

[9] Amiel-Tison C., Korobkin R. and Esque-Vaucouloux M. T. Neck extensor hypertonia: a clinical sign of insult of the central nervous system of the newborn. *Early Hum. Dev., 1*, 181, 1977.

4

COMPLEMENTARY NEUROMOTOR EXAMINATION: Early Affirmation of Normalcy

Goals and Basic Theory

The complementary neuromotor examination (CNME) of the newborn and young infant is used to expand and enrich the findings of the classical neuromotor examination. The goal is to identify infants who do not have CNS dysfunction soon after birth and to predict good outcome in both motor and cognitive function as early as possible during the first 3 or 4 months of life. Therefore, this examination is particularly important in newborns at high risk for neurological problems secondary to perinatal difficulties. We are convinced that it is not possible to judge the integrity of the CNS by using "cold" techniques that do not solicit the personal participation of the infant, even though the infant might be in an optimal state as in Prechtl's states 3 or 4. For this reason the CNME cannot be reduced to two or three dynamic manipulations.

This is a totally different clinical approach from the basic neuromotor examination described in the last chapter. It will show the parents the competence of their newborn and the integrity of his CNS. In order to draw these conclusions the CNME anticipates the development of the infant. The examiner must create situations of observation during which the infant can be led through a series of interactional and motor performances that demonstrate the absence of major handicap.

No score is used to interpret the results. Indeed a basic premise of this examination is to refuse to give scores to the infants. Either the response of the infant will appear natural, identical to those of an older baby, or the results are not clear, in which case no judgment should be made. The evaluation will subsequently be repeated as many times as necessary in order to obtain satisfactory results. The responses to this examination are completely dependent on the conditions of observation; when the infant's responses are not satisfactory it is more often a result of suboptimal examination conditions rather than problems with the infant per se.

The conditions of the CNME are not very difficult to maintain, particularly when the examiner understands their importance. The conditions are based on changing the neuromotor behavior of the newborn and young infant that is most strongly affected by the physiological *impotence of the neck.* Abrupt movements of the head provoke a parasitical movement of the upper extremities, the Moro reflex, and an interruption of attention that affects all sensorial and motor activity. Evidently this dependence disappears as the infant grows older. However, it is possible to anticipate the development of the infant by *artificially creating head control.* The neck is fixed manually throughout the examination; the infant is maintained in sitting position or in a semireclining position as on a divan, called the *Récamier.**

Within several minutes the infant's contact and motor behavior changes; his movements resemble those of an older infant whose motor activity has already lost its reflex character. This phenomenon has been described as "liberated motor activity" [1].

We have also found that in a well-controlled situation, with the infant seated on a bench as if behind a desk, the infant can show the capacity to grasp an object intentionally (Fig. 4-1). This is not a frequent result and requires an examination that is too long to be used routinely in the CNME. However, the existence of this ability shows that there is voluntary motor activity of the newborn and young infant, and it can be used for early affirmation that there is no major motor handicap.

Intentional motor activity is the most reliable way to affirm the integrity of motor pathways. At the age of walking, one can simply observe the baby walking in all directions. Even before the ability to walk appears, observing how the infant maintains the sitting position, or reaches for an object, or uses the lower extremities to reestablish equilibrium—all show normal motor organization. "Normalcy" is not a clearcut notion in a young infant, particularly before 3 months of age, because motor performance cannot be elicited without preparation. The examiner must begin by liberating the motor ability of the infant before making any interpretation, and must bring the infant into a state

*In the first half of the nineteenth century Madame Récamier had a renowned literary salon where she received the notable writers and poets of the era, semireclined on a divan. Such a divan became known as a Récamier, after her.

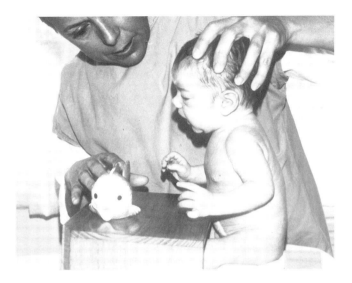

Fig. 4-1 Liberated motor activity. Ability to intentionally grasp a toy that he has never seen before.

other than those described by Prechtl before beginning the evaluation. We call this the "liberated state," because the infant has temporarily lost his primary reflex motor activity and is free to communicate and free to move. Having attained the liberated state, the infant must now be led by the examiner to demonstrate his own normalcy. The specific motor exercises the examiner chooses among the innate motor pathways [2] and the specific dynamic tests [3,4] (described below) are of little importance provided that they lead to a common goal: showing subtle motor ability in the lateral plane, which is early evidence of normalcy (well before 3 months corrected age). Can the infant be led to sit from the lying position (Figs. 4-2 and 4-3)? Can he lean on his outstretched arm and progressively straighten on one side (Fig. 4-4)? Is he capable of straightening his head on his shoulder when he is destabilized and at the same time can he use his leg as a counterweight to reestablish his equilibrium (Fig. 4-5)? The observer will use sufficient maneuvers to show the integrity of the CNS, that is, to demonstrate the intentional and voluntary participation of the infant to straighten his head and trunk against gravity.

This performance, obtained before the normal age of acquisition, combined with the motor exercises that elicit this performance, constitute the CNME.

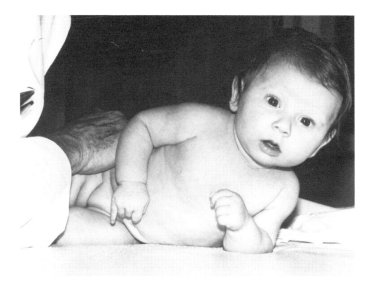

Figs. 4-2 and 4-3 A 3-month-old infant. Will he arrive at the sitting position from the position of lying on his side?

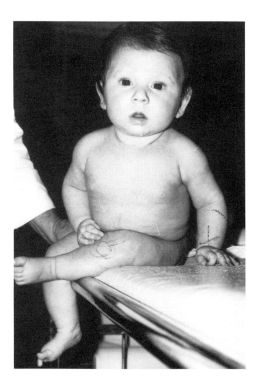

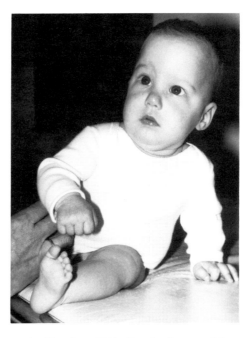

Fig. 4-4 A 1½-month-old infant (GA). Can he lean on his outstretched arm and straighten on his side?

Fig. 4-5 A 2-month-old infant. Can he straighten his head on his shoulder when he loses his balance and at the same time, lift his lower extremity in extension to reestablish equilibrium (reaction of lateral abduction)?

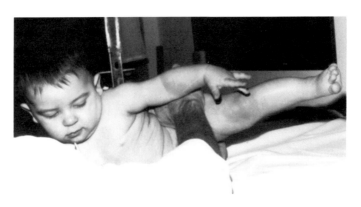

Techniques and Interpretation

The techniques for the CNME are described in the following order: (1) the maneuvers of "debugging" that lead to the *liberated state;* (2) once that state has been attained, the maneuvers that will show motor ability and demonstrate the absence of major CNS dysfunction; and (3) the motor exercises grouped under the term *directed motor activity.*

DEBUGGING

Debugging is the process by which the active participation of the infant is obtained. The infant is brought from his usual state of involuntary and undirected activity to one in which he interacts with the examiner. The examiner makes contact with the infant and maintains it throughout, since any slight period of inattention may affect the infant's motor responses. Another integral part of the debugging process is the temporary suspension of the Moro reflex. The Moro reflex is responsible for the greatest amount of involuntary parasitical movements in the infant up to 3 months of age, at which time reflex motor activity spontaneously disappears. Debugging is accomplished by the combination of several actions.

Calm environment and gentle maneuvers

How is this done? It must be remembered that the Moro reflex is stimulated by abrupt stretching of the muscles of the neck, whether from a rapid movement of the head, movements of the arms, a sudden noise, a bright light, an unexpected manipulation of the infant, or simply jostling of the infant's bed. The examiner must carefully prepare the infant for the evaluation:

See that the examining room is warm.
Take advantage of a period of digestion between two feedings.
Allow few persons around the infant.
Speak in a low voice.
Eliminate any very bright light.

Why attempt to abolish the Moro reflex? This reflex interferes with most of the motor activity that can be used to affirm normal neuromotor function in the young infant. It is associated with involuntary parasitical movements that interrupt all the activity of the arms; it facilitates crying and suspends the attention and availability of the infant. In fact the Moro reflex can return at any moment during the examination, even after several minutes of preparation. Therefore the examiner must remain vigilant and avoid interruptions. If control of the infant is inadvertently lost, it is essential to suspend the examination for 1 or 2 minutes and begin again when a calm environment has been restored.

Manual fixation of the neck

This is the first action the examiner will take upon touching the infant. How is it accomplished? The infant is facing the examiner and is maintained in a semisitting position on the examining table. His head must be fixed by a hand that is placed behind the neck. The infant must be calm and must be in contact with the examiner. He is first brought gently either to a lateral recumbent position or to a vertical sitting position. The examiner gently raises a hand behind the infant's head to hold the temporal region (Fig. 4-6). The examiner's elbow is firmly

Fig. 4-6 Liberated motor activity: starting position (day 10). Examiner holds infant's neck and head firmly with one hand. Examiner's elbow is placed on table.

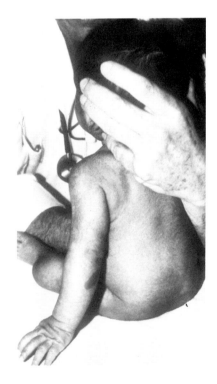

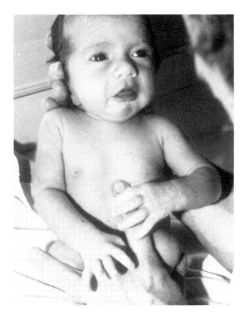

Fig. 4-7   Liberated motor activity: starting position (day 8). Infant manipulates examiner's fingers. Movements are similar to those seen in older infants.

against the table and his or her forearm is behind the infant's shoulder without supporting the back.

Why is this fixation of the neck fundamental? Because when it is not present, the infant loses all ability to communicate with the examiner. He cannot fix his attention or control the movements of his upper extremities. However, when the neck is fixed for several moments the anticipation of development begins (Fig. 4-7); the infant reacts as if he had natural head control, which would not normally occur until ~3 months corrected age. The infant's motor activity can be considered liberated from the involuntary reflex motor activity that interferes with all spontaneous movements.

Soliciting sensorial ability and interaction

The examiner must talk to the infant continuously in a soft voice to capture his attention without startling him. He or she must maintain eye-to-eye contact with the infant to obtain continuous visual communication (Fig. 4-8). With his or her free hand the examiner continuously caresses the infant's skin and applies gentle pressure to the in-

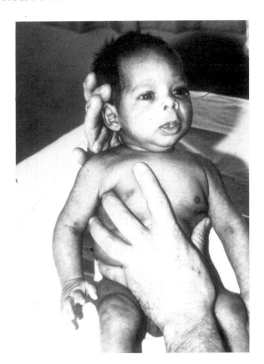

Fig. 4-8   Liberated motor activity: starting position (day 18). Examiner provides countersupport by placing one hand on infant's abdomen.

fant's muscles to stimulate the cutaneous and proprioceptive senses, without startling the infant.

The reason for maintaining this state of sensorial communication is that it is the basis for more elaborate communication, which leads to contact between the examiner and the infant. It is essential to obtain this state, because it plays an active role in the motor exercises described below.

Controlling the position of the trunk

Several different maneuvers are used to control the position of the infant's trunk along with that of the head during the different parts of the examination.

FIRST STAGE: SIMPLE SITTING POSTURE.   The infant is seated on the examining table without back support and the trunk is held vertically. With a newborn or very young infant (who is still "floppy"), the examiner can hold the neck with one hand and place the other hand

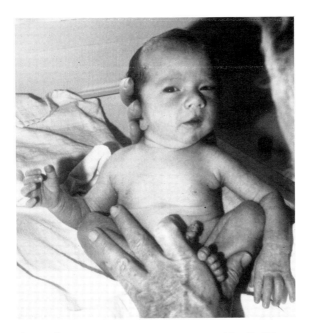

Fig. 4-9   Liberated motor activity: starting position (day 8). The examiner can bring the lower extremities into flexion and gently rock them.

open on the abdomen to give counterpressure. If necessary the index finger can provide light support to the chin if the face tends to fall forward. If the infant is moving his legs, the examiner can lower his or her hand on the abdomen, place the legs in a hyperflexed position, and gently rock them to stimulate them to relax (Fig. 4-9). This control of the position of the infant's head and trunk by the examiner's two hands must not result in total immobility. Instead guided movements of low amplitude and constant speed, which the infant will not resist, are used to avoid stretching of the cervical muscles. To do this the examiner moves his or her hand in a sort of continuously vibrating fashion. It is also recommended to impart slight pistonlike movements to the head, without stimulating a "reflex" response. The joint action of the two hands comforts the infant and is therefore indispensable to the establishment of interaction.

SECOND STAGE: SITTING ON A BENCH.   The infant is seated on a bench placed on the examining table. This is an optional stage that the examiner can use to evaluate the straightening ability of the infant or to examine his sensorial availability and his capacity to grasp intention-

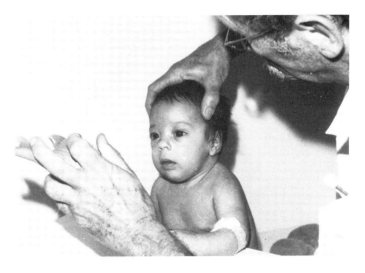

Fig. 4-10 Liberated motor activity: second observational situation (1 month). Only the head is fixed by the examiner. The infant's gaze is fixed on a toy.

Fig. 4-11 Infant of 6 weeks. Position called *Récamier*—like on a divan!

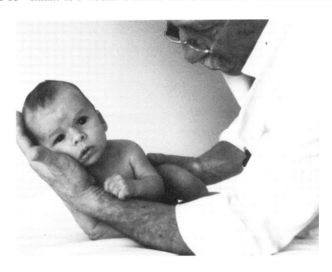

ally a toy on a desk in front of him. The height of the bench is adapted to the size of the infant so that his thighs will be horizontal and his feet will be in front of the bench on the examining table. The examiner continues to hold the head, and instead of remaining directly across from the infant, stays slightly to the side. He or she breaks visual contact with the infant for a moment, so that the infant can become interested in either another observer or an object (a toy) (Fig. 4-10). The infant is not kept immobile; the pistonlike movements of the neck continue, accompanied by subtle swaying movements of the body. It is important to be certain that the axis of the head and the trunk *remain aligned*. It should be noted that at the end of the examination when the examiner relaxes his or her hold, the liberated state persists for a short time. The reflex motor activity of the upper extremities, usually stimulated by movements of the head, is temporarily suppressed.

THIRD STAGE: THE RÉCAMIER POSITION. Beginning in the semisitting position with the neck fixed, the infant is gently placed in a lateral decubitus position (right or left side), with the examiner's hand maintaining control of the infant's head to avoid abrupt movements, even slight ones. The head, aligned with the trunk, leans on the examiner's hand as if the infant were reclining on a divan (Fig. 4-11). There are several specifications: the axis of the head and trunk must be in the same plane; the legs are kept flexed by the examiner's free hand, which can be gradually withdrawn. The infant's lower arm must be placed so that it is perpendicular to the table, with the elbow at a 90-degree angle and the forearm leaning on the table; the hand may be open or closed (Fig. 4-12). The other arm, which is above the body, should be flexed and lying on the trunk; it will begin to move slowly. This hand is open and in many cases moves toward the face of the examiner and often tries to grasp it (Fig. 4-13).

The interactive state that was attained in the sitting position must be reestablished and may even be reinforced, since this reclining position is often more comfortable for the infant. The examiner continuously works at sensorial communication, visual and auditory, and also gently changes the force of the hand supporting the infant's head. After minor resistance this encourages the infant to allow passive support. Progressively, with enhanced interaction, the postural control of the head will change. The examiner will feel an active reinforcement of the lateral muscles of the neck. This reaction of the infant demonstrates the infant's participation and communication. This is the essential benefit of the Récamier position—to avoid abrupt movements of the head and their consequence. It places the infant in the plane of the table, from

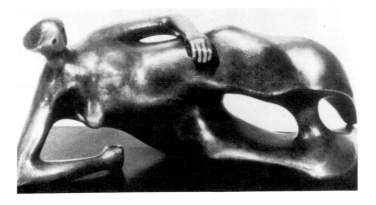

Fig. 4-12 Sculpture by Henry Moore, Galerie Maeght, Paris. The age of individual may be different, but the position is identical to the one used for infants in the CNME.

Fig. 4-13 Liberated motor activity: Récamier position (2 months). The upper extremity that is above falls forward on the infant's trunk and moves slowly; the hand stays open, apparently ready to grasp.

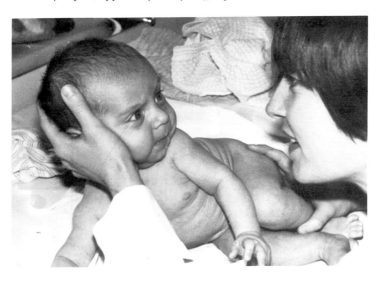

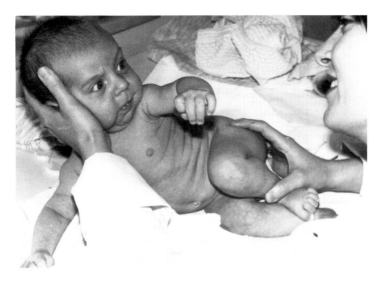

Fig. 4-14 Liberated motor activity: Récamier position (2 months). The examiner will feel the active reinforcement of tone of the muscles of the neck; this is the time to place the body in the plane of the table and prepare the head for its role as "starter."

which the motor evaluation begins, and prepares the infant's head to play its role as the "starter"—that is, to begin straightening against gravity during the dynamic maneuvers that follow (Fig. 4-14).

THE LIBERATED STATE

The term liberated state describes the sensorimotor availability obtained by simultaneous auditory, visual, cutaneous, and proprioceptive stimulation on the one hand, and by the temporary suppression of the effects of the physiological impotence of the neck on the other. This state begins in the first 3 or 4 minutes of the examination. At first, the infant fights against the force that is holding him. He moves around making jerking movements of the trunk or the head. He passes from state 2 to state 5 with no apparent reason. But this situation does not last. The infant's interest in the examiner grows, and a state unlike those described by Prechtl ensues. It is called a *state of communication*, because the infant is actually communicating with the examiner. There is a progression observed in this state. Initially the communication is purely sensorial, as indicated by the absence of crying or agita-

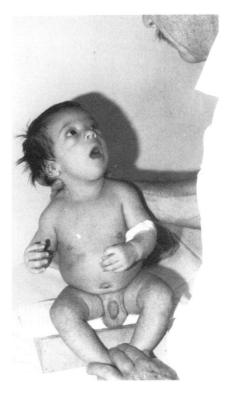

Fig. 4-15　Liberated motor activity: second observational situation (1 month). Contact is obtained: the infant begins taking a true personal interest in the examiner.

tion by the infant. He seems to be listening to the continuous speaking of the examiner, his eyes following the movements of the examiner's head, which is just in front of the infant. Communication may not go farther than this *stage of sensorial availability*, particularly when the infant is very young. Often, but not always, the situation progresses to a state of *true contact*. This state is easy to recognize, in that the infant literally searches out the examiner. He fixes his regard on the examiner; he is almost mesmerized, listening to what the examiner is saying, making imitative movements with his tongue and mouth, and attempting to respond and to smile, as seen by the change of expression in his face (Fig. 4-15). At the same time there is a change in behavior; the arms stop moving in stereotypical obligatory ways. Initially they are raised to the shoulders at the least indication of a struggle. Little by little these movements occur less frequently and less forcefully. Soon the arms go down to the trunk (Fig. 4-16). The hands open and the

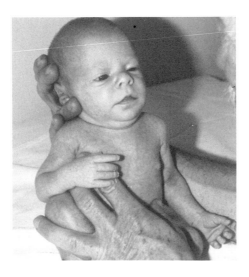

Fig. 4-16 Liberated motor activity: starting position (day 12). Infant's upper extremities are relaxed; hands are open.

Fig. 4-17 Liberated motor activity: second observational situation (day 14). If infant is placed in sitting position, dorsal kyphosis will disappear after several minutes.

Fig. 4-18 Liberated motor activity: second observational situation (day 12). Infant grasps object but releases this hold when object is lifted. Other hand is extended.

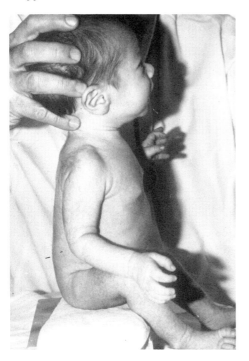

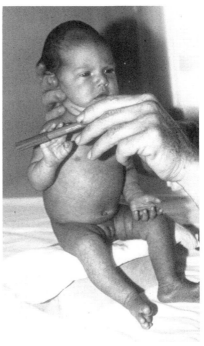

111

fingers spread. Sometimes the thumb stays folded on the palm. Finally, without specific stimulation, there are a few spontaneous movements. They are slow and of limited amplitude but appear smooth and coordinated like the movements of an older infant.

When the infant is seated on a bench the liberated state is even clearer. The trunk, which until then needed support, straightens more and more, and after 5 to 10 minutes physiological kyphosis completely disappears (Fig. 4-17). The arms are completely relaxed. The grasping reflex disappears. An object placed in the hand provokes only a slight response by the fingers that is not firm and stops as soon as the object is taken away (Fig. 4-18). The same phenomenon of inhibition is seen for the Moro reflex and the tonic neck reflex. Movement or rotation of the head provokes no motor response of the upper extremities.

The liberated state is obtained more easily and rapidly in the Récamier position than in the sitting position on a bench. In 4 to 5 minutes the infant becomes *free to communicate and act.* The examiner has the definite impression of creating a "window" through the primary motor activity across which he or she can establish contact that goes beyond the sensorial level. In effect if the infant is comfortable he establishes an interaction of regard, smiling, and listening which is evident. Free to communicate and free to have some voluntary motor activity, the infant still has a few spontaneous movements. The examiner must choose this optimal time to enhance the interaction with the infant and guide him to execute changes of position that will make it possible to identify the absence of major motor anomalies.

DIRECTED MOTOR ACTIVITY

Testing of motor activity will begin only when the infant is in the liberated state, in the Récamier position. The goal is early demonstration of motor pathways. The infant, having temporarily lost his primary motor activity, is in theory free to act, but it is clear that at this early age he lacks the maturation and learned experience to act completely alone. He has neither the desire nor the initiative to change his position, nor does he have the strength to counteract gravity. The examiner must assist him, selecting those dynamic motor tests that will show the integrity of the motor pathways and at the same time give the infant enough opportunity to act on his own so that his active participation is not in doubt. While directing the infant in these motor exercises the examiner gives minimal support to the parts of the infant's body that he would have difficulty moving against gravity on his own.

The choice of the motor exercises comes from the experience of following infants at risk for neurological problems of perinatal origin. It involves demonstrating motor responses that an infant even several months older would never be able to perform correctly. It must be emphasized that the newborn and young infant have a very rich motor repertory [5]. They are capable of executing movements identical to those of an older child or an adult placed in the same situation, as if at birth motor function were already programmed. The only difference is that for the newborn the examiner initiates the response and supports the infant until the end of the exercise. The most reliable technique to demonstrate motor function is straightening in the *lateral plane* when it is executed according to a strict protocol. This involves two exercises: (1) the straightening of the head and the trunk in the process of an intentional effort called *lateral support* and (2) the straightening in abduction of the lower extremity as a result of a chain reaction on one side of the body called the *reaction of lateral abduction* (RLA). It is also helpful to use a series of exercises of turning of the body to each side led by either the head or the lower limbs. This is particularly valuable when the RLA cannot be obtained.

Lateral straightening of the head and body resulting from intentional effort: lateral support

This test is not new, but the liberated state has facilitated its execution and has made the interpretation easier when looking for normal motor function. The movements will evolve according to a fixed motor scheme that will be more or less complete depending on the age of the infant and on the active role he plays to work against gravity.

The starting point is the Récamier position. Very shortly after obtaining the liberated state, before the infant becomes fatigued or cries, maintaining intense contact, the infant is gently placed in a complete lateral decubitus position. The head rests on the examining table, which should be supple, so as not to make the infant uncomfortable. The examiner places one hand on the hip of the infant and gently applies pressure (Fig. 4-19). This pressure initiates the straightening of the upper part of the body, which results in the head being raised. The lower extremities should be placed at the edge of the table in such a way that the legs will be hanging over the edge of the table if he raises himself to a full sitting position at the end of the maneuver. With the other hand the examiner can give a little support with his or her second and third fingers in the fold of the flexed elbow of the upper arm.*

---

*When the infant is in the lateral or lateral decubitus position, two types of terminology are used to indicate the extremity above or below the axis of the body: *upper* or *lower* arm or leg, and arm or leg *underneath* or *on top* of the body.

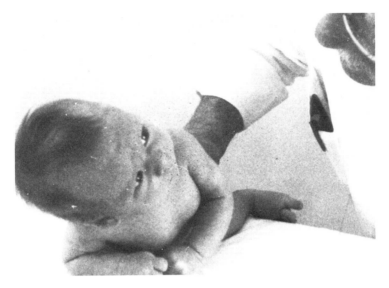

Fig. 4-19   Directed motor activity: lateral support (6 weeks). The examiner leans on the infant's hip as if gently pushing it toward the table, but maintains the state of contact continuously.

This is not meant to provide support to the infant but simply a fixed point against which the infant can rise.

By a force and a will that comes from the infant himself, the head straightens more and more, and the contraction of the shoulder muscles supports the infant on the table. If the young infant is not actively participating, the postural reaction may stop at this point. By contrast, when the infant is actively participating, the maneuver continues to completion; the straightening of the head is followed by the progressive straightening of the trunk, which may end with the infant in a sitting position. The position of the lower arm changes with the amount of straightening of the body. First the infant leans on the forearm with the elbow flexed, then with the elbow at a 90-degree angle, and finally on the hand, with the elbow extended and the fist open or closed. Support on the forearm increases with age and is complete before 3 months corrected age. These maneuvers must be repeated several times with the active participation of the infant, before concluding that these straightening abilities are absent or insufficient (Figs. 4-20 to 4-22).

What is the significance of this ability in a young infant? We do not as yet have statistics on long-term outcome, but our personal experience leads us to conclude that the overall motor and relational behavior demonstrates a sound central organization, incompatible with cerebral damage. We think that such responses have important significance that implies intact motor organization and the possibility to obtain intense contact with the surroundings. How is it possible to imagine a cerebral lesion in an infant of several weeks who grabs your eyeglasses with gusto (Fig. 4-23)? As we have come to understand the great competence of the newborn, his power of adaptation, and his ability to interact (seen most intensely with his mother), we feel an early assessment of the psychomotor state is possible through the evaluation of motor responses and a concomitant state of contact.

Is error of interpretation possible? In order to avoid errors, there must be no interpretation made when the infant is not ready for this clinical approach in either the motor or sensory areas. The attempts can be renewed many times, as long as the infant tolerates it. Erroneous results can be attributed to peripheral anomalies of the muscles of the neck. The following precautions are therefore necessary:

1. Palpate the lateral muscles to ensure that there is neither a hematoma nor a tendinous retraction that could explain asymmetric straightening. An easy raising of the head can be a simple passive straightening from a muscle that is too short (Fig. 4-24). Inversely, insufficient force of straightening on the side opposite from such a shortening has no neurological significance.

2. Ensure that the head and the axis of the trunk are aligned. This may be difficult to obtain when the extensor muscles of the neck (essentially the *trapezius*) are *shortened* (Fig. 4-25). A falsely inadequate response may occur if during the maneuver the infant turns his face up and it then appears that his head is not able to straighten; a falsely positive response can occur in the opposite situation, if the infant looks downward toward the plane of the table.

3. Do not assume that the trapezius muscles are short without evaluating the specific case: why would these muscles have shortened? Also, do not make any assumptions without having attempted the maneuver of lateral straightening several times. Shortening of the posterior muscles of the neck can be seen with (1) a continuous or preferential position of ventral decubitus, (2) an iatrogenic shortening secondary to the maintenance of the head in hyperextension in the course of intensive care, (3) opisthotonos of neurological origin, observed particularly as a transient anomaly in high-risk newborns [6], and (4) as the first sign of a cerebral malformation, particularly of the posterior fossa.

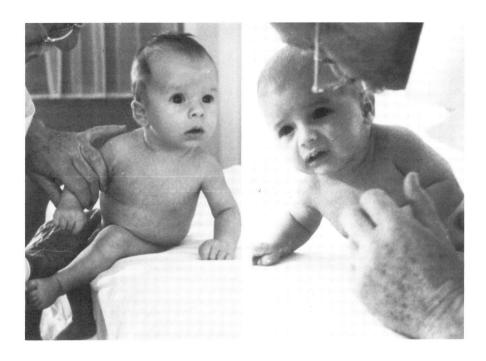

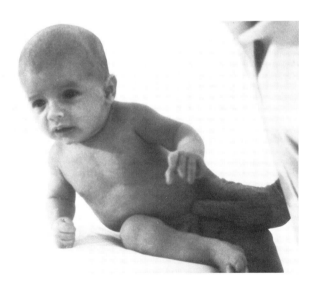

Figs. 4-20 to 4-22 Directed motor activity: lateral support (two infants at 6 weeks). The infant has used his own force to complete straightening. The examiner has not pulled on the arm, but only offers a point of support.

116

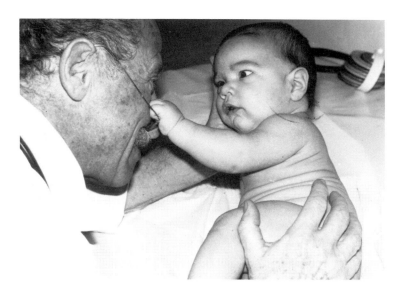

Fig. 4-23 A 2-month-old infant—who takes off your glasses.

Fig. 4-24 Directed motor activity: lateral support (6 weeks). Impossible to evaluate because the lateral muscles of the neck on the left side are too short.

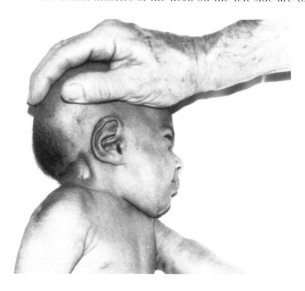

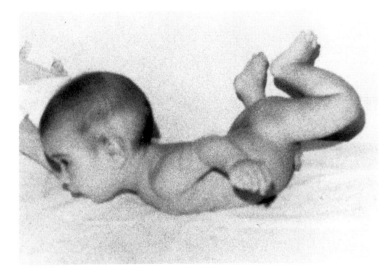

Fig. 4-25   Retraction of the trapezius muscles resulting in the "glider" position (6 weeks).

The significance of lateral straightening as a voluntary effort by the infant is such that if its absence or asymmetry is suspected, there must be repeated evaluations at short intervals, and transfontanellar ultrasound and tomographic studies are indicated. In all cases of confirmed *asymmetry*, the examiner must not only carefully compare the two sides of the body so as not to miss a hemihypertrophy that could explain an asymmetric response in an infant who maintains a dorsal decubitus position slightly rolled on the "hypotrophic side," but also compare the tone and force of movements in the liberated state, which may reveal an asymmetry resulting from a cerebral lesion that would evolve as a spastic hemiplegia later in childhood.

Reaction of lateral abduction of the hip

The RLA is a postural reaction that provokes a chain of muscular contractions on one side of the body from the head to the feet, at the end of which frank abduction of the hip is observed. Under specific conditions the result is a lateral straightening of the lower extremity, which is raised in extension against gravity. Twenty years of experience with many infants, both normal and with cerebral motor handicap, have shown that this reaction is always absent in children with a motor handicap, even in the newborn period before the handicap can be clin-

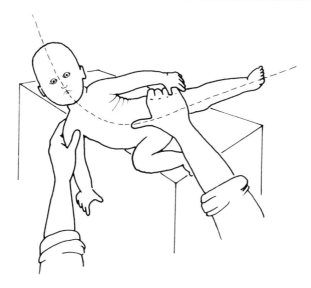

Fig. 4-26   Schematic drawing of the RLA of the hip (A. Grenier's maneuver).

ically confirmed [4]. Originally it represented a *reaction of equilibra-tion* such as that observed in an older child sitting on the edge of a table, legs hanging, who is jostled from the right or left without a chance to use the hands for balance; the child will straighten his head to the side, and will raise the lower extremity on the side opposite from the jolt in a effort to regain balance. As long as the position is strictly maintained (see below), the raising of the lower extremity can only be a result of the abduction of the hip (Fig. 4-26). Everything occurs as if there is an equilibrium established between the force of straightening of the head and the force of straightening of the lower extremity raised against gravity. Active contractions start in the lateral muscles of the neck and traverse one side of the body without interruption; they pro-ceed to the hip, thigh, the knee in extension, the leg, and then the foot, which is at a right angle to the axis of the lower extremity. It is the response as a whole that demonstrates intact motor organization. Once it has appeared, it remains for life (Fig. 4-27). It is clinically evident at around the eighth month, when the infant has a well -organized reaction of equilibration. It was not formerly known whether this ability to react against a force to regain equilibrium was present in an infant <3 months old. It is by first reinforcing the straightening reaction of the head of a very young infant that the demonstration of this ability in the newborn and young infant is made possible.

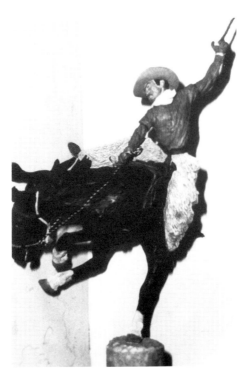

Fig. 4-27 Reaction of lateral abduction by a cowboy (John Wayne himself) and his horse, during a rodeo. (Western Museum of Fame, Oklahoma City, photo by Paul Toubas.)

TECHNIQUE OF ELICITING THE REACTION OF LATERAL ABDUCTION.

Starting position. The infant is placed in the lateral decubitus position on a table, facing the examiner. His head must not be leaning on the table; the lower extremity that is underneath is maintained in *flexion* so as not to participate in the reaction. The other lower extremity is placed and maintained in *extension*. This position is fundamental to obtain a RLA and it must be maintained throughout the maneuver.

Beginning of the RLA. The head plays the role of starter. In order to obtain the reaction, a series of lateral straightening movements of the head must be provoked (the technique depends on the age of the infant). It is as a result of one of these movements of the head that the reaction is set off.

Development of the RLA. The examiner must clearly observe the straightening of the head and the chain of contractions that follow along

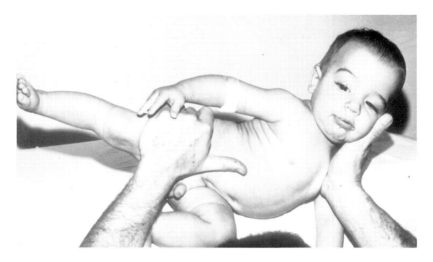

Fig. 4-28 Reaction of lateral abduction: final result. The lower extremity lifts in abduction without flexion of the thigh or the hip. The infant tolerates the maneuver without crying and without movements of defense (hand open, face relaxed).

Fig. 4-29 Reaction of lateral abduction. Development of the reaction can be seen in the lateral straightening of the head, the chain of contractions of the trunk, the extension of the lower extremity, and the position of the foot (dorsal flexion, pointed toward the examiner).

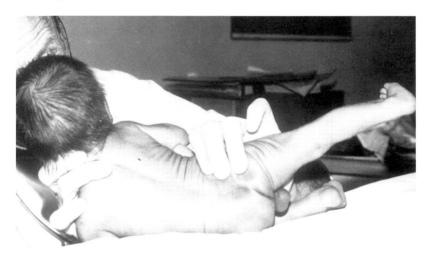

the body. They start from the neck, travel down the trunk, which curves inward laterally and reach the pelvis; they then descend along the thigh and leg in extension, ending in the foot, which is in dorsiflexion with the toes pointing toward the examiner.

Results. Once the position of the extremity that is underneath is correct, abduction of the hip is observed. The whole extremity lifts against gravity as a result of abduction of the hip (Figs. 4-28 and 4-29).

CONDITIONS TO FOLLOW.   The following conditions are important for the successful completion of the RLA.   *First condition: alignment of the axes of the extremities and the trunk.*   In order to be sure that it is only the abductors of the hip that raise the upper leg, the thigh must be in perfect extension on the pelvis. In other words, the axes of the extremities and the trunk must be in perfect alignment. It is helpful to imagine a line from the ear to the lateral maleolus that is followed by the lateral side of the hip and the knee (Fig. 4-30). If there is not such an alignment, the maneuver is not reliable and the response is false. In effect, when there is the slightest degree of flexion of the thigh on the hip, it is not the abductors that raise the leg but rather an action of the flexors of the hip. A "false abduction" will give false results. This alignment of the axes of the trunk and the lower

Fig. 4-30 Reaction of lateral abduction. Alignment of the heel–ear axis; correct position of the foot, with the toes pointed toward the examiner.

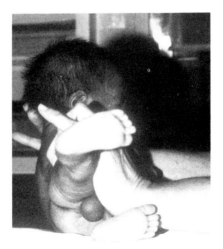

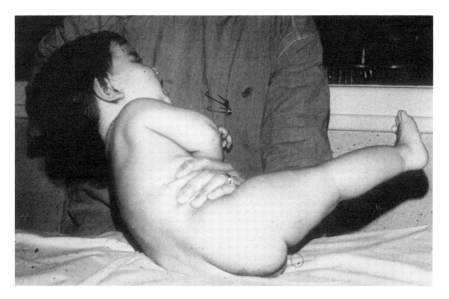

Fig. 4-31 Reaction of lateral abduction. False abduction. The thigh is flexed on the pelvis thereby invalidating the reaction, since it was the flexors of the hip that were activated by the chain of contractions.

extremity must be taken even farther. Any "break" in the alignment, such as flexion of the head, rolling of the trunk, flexion of the hip, flexion of the knee, or external rotation of the foot with the toes pointing upward, will give false results (Fig. 4-31). Any break allows "leakage" of contractions in the flexors of the hip, which interferes with the maneuver. To avoid such errors several specific techniques (described below) are used to maintain the hip in extension throughout the maneuver. These techniques are most important for the very small infant in whom the thigh spontaneously flexes on the pelvis.

Second condition: repetition of lateral movements of head to achieve active postural control. The movement of the head, which plays the role of starter, must be repeated until the infant himself completes the response. The head must straighten on the side; that is, the ear approaches the shoulder without rotation of the neck. The face must remain strictly in the same plane. These movements are obtained in different ways according to the age and the postural abilities of the infant.

1. When the infant is capable of postural control of his head, the examiner bends the trunk without touching the head. The head raises

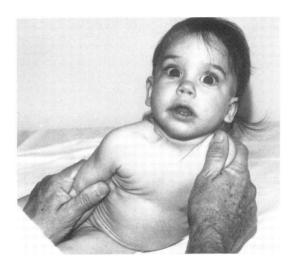

Fig. 4-32 Reaction of lateral abduction. Lateral movements of the head. The infant himself holds his head up, keeping the "line of the eyes" horizontal when the examiner leans him to the side.

spontaneously and maintains this position by repeated contractions, so that the eyes are maintained on an imaginary horizontal line (Fig. 4-32). These are the straightening efforts that provoke the RLA.

2. When the infant is unable to straighten his head independently, the examiner must bend the trunk and hold the head with his or her hand. This hand is used to provoke a series of rapid straightening and relaxing movements of the neck (Figs. 4-33 and 4-34) throughout the maneuver. Often this will result in an active contraction and will set off the RLA. The ability of lateral straightening of the neck exists soon after birth, just like posterior straightening when the infant is in the ventral position and anterior straightening in the "pull-to-sit maneuver." However, this lateral straightening ability is less well known and is seen only when the infant is in a lateral position and loses his balance.

Third condition: active support of the body. However the infant is held, all of the infant's weight must not be in the examiner's hands. The examiner should feel a relaxation in his or her support of the tonic body and should continuously be adjusting the contractions. To facilitate the maneuver we suggest placing the infant on the edge or the corner of a table with the head and trunk directed over the side, the lower hip acting as the point of contact with the table. This attention

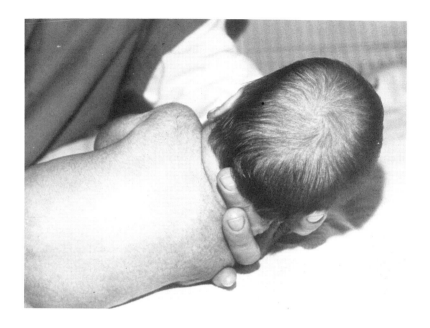

Figs. 4-33 and 4-34 Reaction of lateral abduction. Lateral movements of the head. The infant cannot straighten his head laterally on his own; the examiner initiates a series of rapid lateral straightening movements.

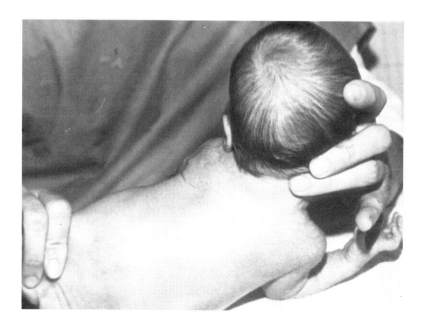

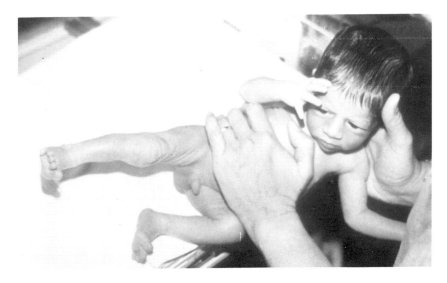

Fig. 4-35 Reaction of lateral abduction. Flexion of the lower extremity that is underneath. This position is essential to avoid confusing the RLA with a defensive straightening of the body.

to position is essential for the infant to attempt straightening against gravity, an outcome that is essential to set off the RLA.

Fourth condition: nonparticipation of upper extremities. The infant must not use his hands at any time during the maneuver, either to hold the examiner or to lean on the table. Use of the hands will eliminate all attempts at straightening and will abolish the extension of the trunk and lower extremity.

Fifth condition: maintenance of lower leg in flexion. The lower extremity that is underneath must be maintained in flexion so that it will not participate in the motor response. This precaution prevents the confusion of an active extension of the lower extremity (part of a simple reaction of defense) with the RLA. It also allows for an increase of force in the involved extremity when it is raised against gravity (Fig. 4-35).

Sixth condition: good general examination conditions. As for all parts of the neurological examination, it is essential to maintain favorable conditions: alertness, digestion, temperature, and so on. This maneuver does not have to be unpleasant. The infant may cry, but this does not necessarily interfere unless he resists. However, as soon as the infant begins to fight the maneuver must be either suspended until he is calm or postponed until some future date.

Some practical advice is in order here. Depending on the age of the infant, the examiner will encounter various problems in meeting all the conditions. Here are some hints that will be helpful concerning the manner of holding the infant at the beginning of and throughout the maneuver.

For infants ≥ 6 months of age (as in the older child and adult), the RLA can be performed from the position seated on the edge of the table with the legs hanging. At this age the baby absorbs all jostling of his body with reactions of equilibration. The examiner can grasp the baby's arms below the shoulders, preventing the hands from gaining support. The examiner jostles the baby's body to one side. The head straightens, and the leg on the side toward which the body leans is maintained with the knee flexed at the edge of the table, or possibly it is held in flexion by an assistant. The other extremity will rise in extension. Placed this way the baby rests on only one buttock. The examiner then pivots the baby, so that the trunk is suspended in space in front of the table. As a result of this rotation the lower extremity, which was in extension, projects in the plane of the table and raises in abduction each time the examiner relaxes his support. In order for the abduction of the hip to be pure, it is possible with the elbow to hold back the baby's thigh so that it is in complete extension on the hips (Fig. 4-36). Throughout this maneuver the examiner must ensure that the baby's body is always in the same plane; if it is not, abduction of the hip will be false.

In infants <6 months old the RLA begins from the reclining position. The examiner must control the head's movements and ensure that the two lower extremities are positioned correctly. This can be done alone or with an assistant. With one hand the examiner puts the lower leg in flexion and extends the opposite thigh, firmly maintaining the extension. With the other hand, he or she initiates the "starter" movements of the head. The cheek and the ear may be directly supported in the examiner's palm as he or she makes slight movements of lateral flexion (Fig. 4-37), or he or she may hold the lower shoulder (Fig. 4-38), leaving the head suspended, making slight up and down movements. Yet another alternative is to hold the upper arm (Fig. 4-39), leaving the head, the shoulder, and part of the trunk suspended. The examiner may have difficulty extending the hip when the thigh is in very active flexion. An assistant can be called on to take care of the

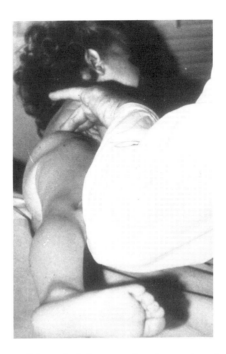

Fig. 4-36 Reaction of lateral abduction after 6 months of age, clinical demonstration. The alignment of the lower extremity is obtained by the examiner pushing the thigh with his elbow. The orientation of the foot and abduction of the hip are perfect.

Fig. 4-37 Reaction of lateral abduction before 6 months of age, clinical demonstration. Examiner holds infant's cheek and ear in his palm while flexing head laterally.

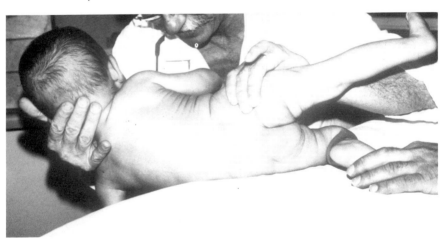

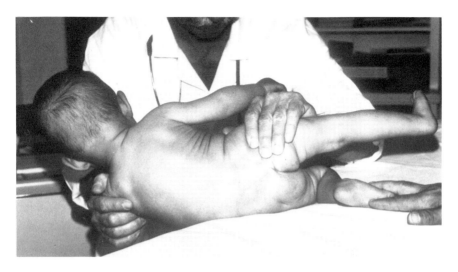

Fig. 4-38 Reaction of lateral abduction before 6 months of age, clinical demonstration. Examiner holds lower shoulder, leaving head suspended over table.

Fig. 4-39 Reaction of lateral abduction before 6 months of age, clinical demonstration. Examiner holds top arm, leaving head and part of trunk suspended over table.

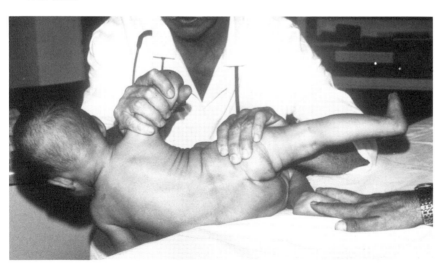

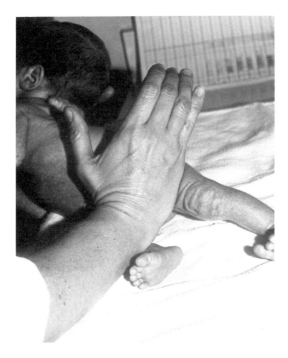

Fig. 4-40 Reaction of lateral abduction before 6 months, clinical demonstration. The examiner must push without forcing the thigh with the palm of his hand to obtain perfect alignment.

Fig. 4-41 Reaction of lateral abduction before 6 months of age, clinical demonstration. Examiner's hand will bridge iliac crest to create countersupport necessary to maintain hip alignment.

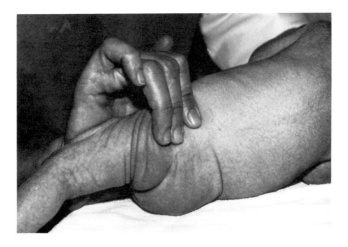

Table 4-1 Principal Neurological Anomalies
Found in 419 Neonates

Anomaly	Number of cases
Hypotonia	87
Hypertonia	66
Modified primary reflexes	20
Hyperexcitability	14
Insufficient postural control	38
Asymmetry	17
Poor contact	25
Miscellaneous	152
TOTAL	419

lower leg, which must be held totally flexed, and to assure that the infant does not lean on his hand and develop a force of straightening that would falsify the reaction. With hands free the examiner can ensure perfect extension of the upper leg. He or she must push the thigh with a palm, without forcing, to arrive at a perfect alignment. This is accomplished by bending the fingers around the iliac crest to give slight but firm counterpressure, making a bridge (Figs. 4-40 and 4-41) that will still allow the lower extremity to raise itself in abduction when the dynamic response occurs.

LONG-TERM SIGNIFICANCE OF THE RLA.   We have not as yet done a controlled prospective study; however, we can provide some data on the retrospective analysis of results of the "unselected" population of our outpatient consultations at Bayonne, France. From 1974 to 1979 we followed 419 children in whom the RLA was attempted and for whom we obtained information on motor development. These 419 children, seen for diverse reasons, were all at high risk for neurological problems as they all had anomalies on the classical neurological examination. These anomalies were an indication for the use of the RLA maneuver (Table 4-1).

The results of the RLA are indicated on Table 4-2. The RLA was absent in 35 children throughout their development; 18 of these 35 have a cerebral motor handicap, that is, 4.6% of the population studied. Early reeducation before age 1 year was started for 13 of the 18. The 17 other children did not have a cerebral motor handicap. The reasons for the absence of the RLA in these 17 children were as follows: congenital hip dysplasia in 6 cases, a subdural effusion without motor sequelae after puncture in 4 cases, and unknown in 7 cases.

Table 4-2 Results of Execution of the RLA in 419 Infants:
Outcome at Age 1 Year or Older in Relation to Absence or
Presence of the Reaction

RLA	Number of cases	Neurological state at 1 year or later
Absent	35	18 with cerebral motor handicap
		17 without cerebral motor handicap
Present	384	384 without cerebral motor handicap
TOTAL	419	

ERRORS AND PROBLEMS OF EXECUTION.   In spite of all the technical
descriptions and warnings, which are essential, a number of errors of
interpretation are possible. Without reiterating the possible technical
faults, the difficulty in appreciating abduction must be emphasized. It
must be *visible:* the foot in dorsiflexion must go up and come down
several times to ensure there is no error of interpretation (Figs. 4-42
and 4-43). The abduction must also be felt by the hand placed over the
iliac crest. The sensation of abduction is clear and cannot be wrongly

Figs. 4-42 and 4-43 Reaction of lateral abduction: dorsiflexion. Foot remains
in dorsiflexion and must move up and down several times.

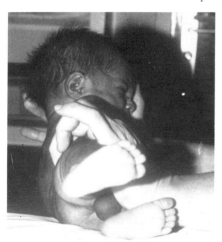
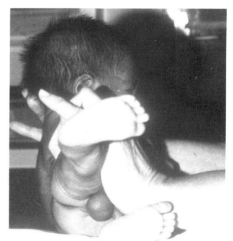

interpreted after it has once been felt. In order for the abduction to be significant, the body must not roll, the lower leg must remain in flexion, and the extremity examined must be in perfect alignment with the extended knee and with the foot, which is pointed toward the examiner. In these conditions the RLA can be considered present without question. However, the infant does not always allow himself to be manipulated without resistance, so that the examiner's attempts are often frustrated. For this reason the maneuver is often reserved for cases in which it is essential to eliminate a CNS lesion. Repeated assessment may be considered of therapeutic value.

Other dynamic tests

There are exercises of turning, straightening, and displacement in all planes of space with the goal of provoking a change in posture. All of these maneuvers belong to the category of directed motor activity, as they are induced and guided by the examiner who can assess the organization, harmony, and control of movements. These maneuvers are used by a number of authors, some of whom have their own protocols for the neuromotor examination [2,3]. It is the tests that involve turning of the body and demonstrate voluntary movements of the lower extremities that are of most interest to us. The significance of these turning movements is not as specific as that of the RLA. However, they are particularly helpful when it is not possible to complete the RLA. The observer should pay careful attention to the movements of the pelvis when the infant begins the movement.

SLOW STEPWISE TURNING OF THE INFANT LYING SUPINE.   Starting from the Récamier position and in a good state of contact, the infant is placed in a supine position. The examiner slowly guides the rotation of the infant starting with the head, which on being turned passively to one side provokes the turning of the rest of the body to roll over. At first there is spirallike movement of the body with only the shoulders following the head; then the trunk and the hips follow, with the lower extremity rising from the table. At this stage the examiner stops the movement of rotation and leaves the infant, half-rotated, in equilibrium resting on his side. Several movements of the head to either side lead the infant to complete the rotation of his head. Then the lower extremity makes several alternating movements of flexion and extension followed by complete rotation of the trunk. The interest of this maneuver is to observe the activity of the upper leg (Figs. 4-44 to 4-46), which flexes in the beginning of the rotation, extends when the infant is on the flank, then flexes again at the hip and the knee so that

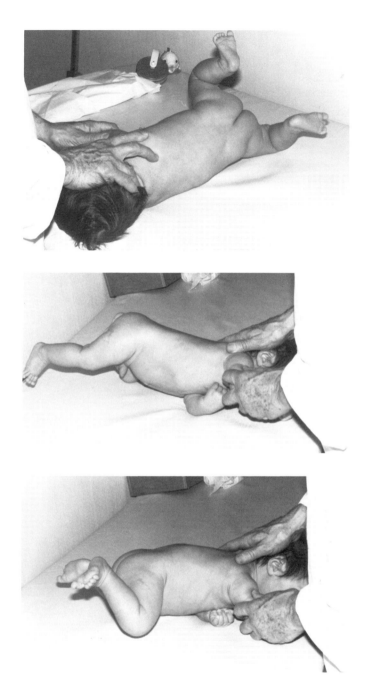

Figs. 4-44 to 4-46 Other dynamic exercises: active turning. If after having begun the turning motion, the examiner stops, the infant will complete the rotation of his body while making organized movements with his lower extremities.

the knee comes to rest on the table next to, but not touching, the other knee.

It is important to avoid a complete turn in one movement with the infant's lower extremities flexed from the beginning to the end of the rotation. Also, the infant should not be startled by an abrupt movement that would stimulate a stretching of the deep muscles of the neck. This in turn could provoke an irrepressible extension of the lower extremities, like in the Moro reflex, which would last throughout the rotation.

To have good participation by the infant it is necessary to prevent crying and all other movements of defense, which would make the lower extremities *move* at the end of the rotation. The responses must be reproducible several times during the same examination.

SUPPORT ON ONE FOOT WITH INFANT IN THE VERTICAL AXIS.   This maneuver involves rotation and straightening of the body, achieved in one continuous movement at constant speed. With the infant lying supine, the feet over the edge of the table, the examiner takes one lower extremity and rolls it over the other. Placing the other hand on the infant's abdomen, the examiner then assists the rotation of the body, which pivots completely on its axis. When rotation is complete, without interrupting the movement the examiner supports the infant's body with one hand placed on the abdomen, as the infant raises his whole body; the other hand holds one lower extremity from the beginning of the maneuver. In this way only one lower extremity is free and as a rule is extended. At the final point of the maneuver the examiner must be able to brush the dorsal aspect of the free foot on the edge of the table so as to provoke a reaction of placement. The foot then applies pressure so that the knee extends and the trunk straightens (Figs. 4-47 to 4-50). The other extremity must be maintained in triple flexion (the heel touching the buttock, the foot in extension and internally rotated), fixed in place by the examiner's fingers.

The examiner should be able to feel the response clearly. In order to avoid confusing the reaction with the simple automatic straightening reaction, the response should not be interpreted before 2 to 3 months of age, that is, not before the disappearance of automatic straightening. Several turns are sometimes necessary for the infant to develop a "forceful" response. If this does not occur, the supporting extremity will be in flexion either throughout the exercise or as soon as the sole of the foot makes contact with the table. When the response is positive, the examiner's hand, which is supporting the abdomen, can feel the force that the infant applies in pushing up from the foot to the hip.

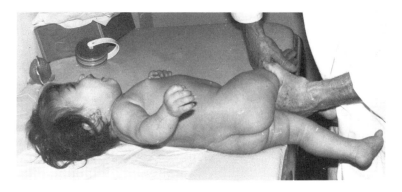

Fig. 4-47 Support on one foot (2½ months). The infant lying supine is rolled over.

Figs. 4-48 and 4-49 Support on one foot (2½ months). The placing reaction is stimulated and obtained.

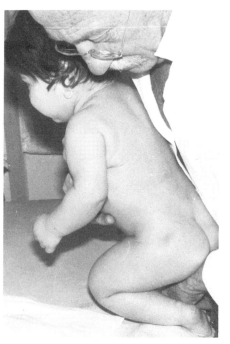 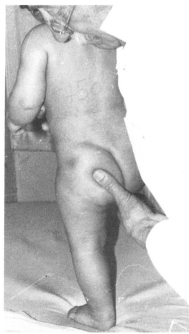

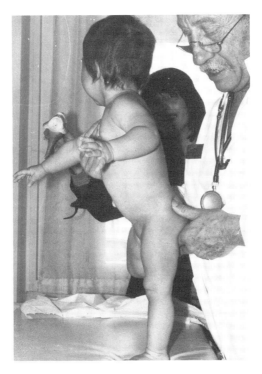

Fig. 4-50 Support on one foot (2½ months). Completion of the maneuver with global straightening.

The examiner's other hand can feel an automatic straightening reaction, which is possible if the infant is at the age when automatic motor activity is just disappearing or if the automatic motor activity is late in disappearing. If the response of the supporting extremity is "reflex" in nature, the examiner feels the flexed extremity straining to extend itself as part of a straightening reaction; in contrast, when the response of the supporting extremity is voluntary the muscles of the other extremity remain relaxed and triple flexion is maintained without any struggle. The quality of motor organization is seen in the infant's force of straightening, that is, his ability to remain upright while supporting himself on one lower extremity. Several movements of circumduction transmitted to the hips from the trunk demonstrate the active contractions of postural adjustment, as would be seen in an older child who stands on one foot.

Place of the Complementary Neuromotor Examination

HISTORY AND EVOLUTION OF IDEAS

The CNME originated in 1970 in the course of following up infants at high risk for cerebral motor sequelae. These outpatient consultations had the difficult task of recognizing handicap as early as possible without confusing it with simple motor delay or reversible neuromotor anomalies. It became clear that the diagnosis of a cerebral motor handicap was not possible in the first months of life—except for severe handicap, which is evident very early. A number of infants were unnecessarily suspected of motor sequelae for several months because of abnormal results on their neurological examinations. It was to decrease the number of "suspects" that the CNME was designed. The goal of the examination was early affirmation of normal motor activity of the lower extremities and from that the prediction of absence of a severe cerebral motor handicap in high-risk infants. To meet this goal the approach is twofold: (1) to devaluate the prognostic significance of most of the early anomalies observed during the first 4 months of life and (2) to increase the value of the newborn's sensorimotor abilities, which are not sufficiently appreciated in the classical neurological examination. These two concepts necessarily led to the development of the first CNME [7]. Initially it involved only the displacement of the body in all planes of space and quickly became dominated by the RLA of the lower extremity. The innovative aspect of the examination has always been that motor responses could only be interpreted if the infant had been well prepared by multiple sensorial stimulation, putting him in a receptive state and in communication with the examiner [4].

Observing the infant for complex motor abilities led to the realization that the performance of the newborn and young infant is dominated by the impotence of the neck. From this observation came the description of "liberated motor activity" [1]. A cohort of 246 infants <8 weeks old (corrected age) were consecutively studied [8]. They were all examined in the sitting position with their neck fixed by the examiner's hand for several minutes. The following observations were made, always in the same sequence:

A lull in reflex motor activity allowing for a state of intense communication with the examiner (97%)
Active support of the trunk and a relaxation of the upper extremities, which moved like those of an older infant (43%)

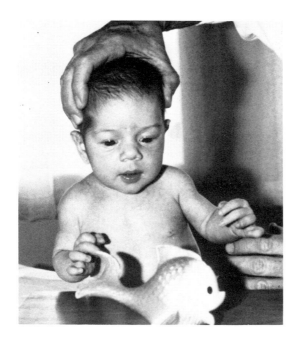

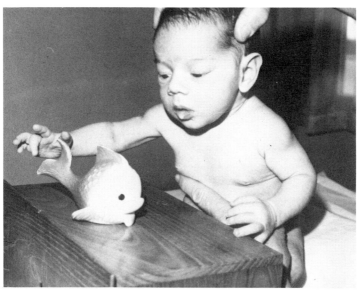

Figs. 4-51 to 4-54 Liberated motor activity (17-day-old infant). See also Figure 4-1. The object is at a distance from the infant and there has been no prior exposure to the object. The arm and hand movements that reach for and grasp the object are never the same from one moment to another; each infant has an individual style but the same intention.

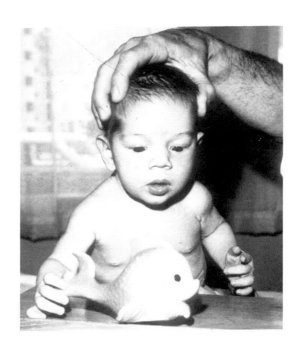

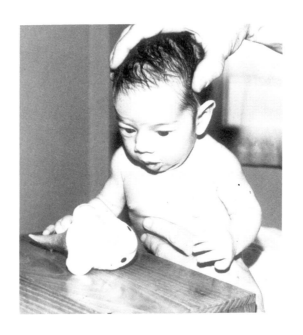

A real interest in an object placed so that the infant intensely fixes his gaze (39%) and grasps and touchs it in an intentional way, repeatedly with precise nonparasitical movements (19%)

The intentional character of the latter response is not in doubt when the object that is grasped is at a distance and there has been no previous contact; this situation differs from the newborn removing a handkerchief placed on his face or caressing the breast of his mother while suckling. In fact in the latter case the infant's hand is relaxed and open as if he were approaching the liberated state; the difference lies in his reaching for an unknown object placed at a distance. The movements of the upper extremities and of the hand that grasps and manipulates the object are never alike from one moment to another or from one infant to another. There seems to exist a predetermined motor ability, a "pattern" in the displacement of the extremity as a whole; however, the intentional activity of the infant can modify this pattern, resulting in movements of variable placement, speed, force, and precision. The hand appears to be under voluntary control and is not acting stereotypically (Figs. 4-51 to 4-54). Therefore, this capacity to grasp an object voluntarily, seen from 14 days of age, corresponds to an ability that already exists in the young infant but is hidden by the global movements set off by the deep reflexes of the neck. These observations led to the hypothesis that liberated motor activity is the precurser of later motor activity of the infant. These observations led us to direct the CNME toward establishing the liberated state [9] as a preliminary to all motor exercises (Figs. 4-51 to 4-54).

IMPORTANCE OF THE CONCEPT OF CONVALESCENCE IN THE HIGH-RISK NEWBORN

The CNME is used from the neonatal period to help the pediatrician conquer a long-standing fear of failure in early recognition of brain damage. The pediatrician who observes neuromotor anomalies in the first months will have to resist the temptation to discuss the possibility of sequelae with the parents. Nothing is certain at such an early age, nor is there any urgency to inform the family of an incurable state. Too many errors are made diagnosing pathology in the 3 or 4 months following discharge from intensive care units. However, there are few situations in which the family of a newborn are already as worried about the future of their child and thus demand a prediction of the outcome. In these cases the notion of convalescence gives the examiner the ability to avoid responding to this pressure too early, providing an "escape" (except in cases of severe encephalopathy). In fact all anomalies of communication, behavior, tone, and/or development can be attributed to the period of convalescence that follows the acute phase of neonatal pathology [10].

This notion of convalescence is not merely an escape, it is a reality. The infant has just temporarily lost precious time during a phase of rapid development. It is completely natural for such an infant to be excessively sleepy or to be hyperexcitable, to have muscular soreness or stiffness, reduced or exaggerated motor responses, or muscle shortening secondary to the restrained positions required for continuous intensive care. The concept of convalescence can be very well understood by the families when explained in this way by the examiner. It extends for a period that begins at the discharge from the intensive care unit and lasts an average of 3 or 4 months. The parents would prefer that it be totally out of the realm of medicine, reserved for their interaction with the infant. There must be complete investment by the family in the infant whether he is handicapped or not, and there should be no development of pejorative feelings that could greatly damage the familial interaction.

This convalescence acts as a break between birth and the recognition of a possible handicap and can be used by the examiner to look for normalcy. Convalescence begins during the hospitalization. The examination can be progressive, spread out over several days, and if possible should be done in the parents' presence. Initially it is enough to put the infant in a state of wakefulness and attention. A little later the motor performances will be solicited. This part of the examination can be done by a physiotherapist who is part of the neonatal team. The examination can be used to establish a link between the mother and infant, and to promote the identification of the newborn as an individual. When the parents are aware that the examiner is looking for "normalcy," they readily return for follow-up visits. In this way very few infants are lost to follow-up. With this understanding of the concept of convalescence, any variation from normal observed during the first 4 months of life will not be considered as abnormal until there is subsequent confirmation.

COMPLEMENTARITY WITH THE CLASSICAL NEUROLOGICAL EXAMINATION

Several differences stand out when the characteristics of the CNME are compared to those of the classical neurological examination.

1. The assessment of motor activity is performed while the infant is in a privileged state of communication. This preliminary point is fundamental. The term liberated state is used to define a specific state that is completely different from Prechtl's five states; this specific state is the result of both manual fixation of the neck and sustained sensorial communication.

2. The CNME uses motor maneuvers that are not part of the repertory of the classical neurological examination. The classical examination gives a clear idea of development but is restricted to the current developmental level of the infant; it does not anticipate future acquisitions. It is often limited to primary motor activity and muscular extensibility and therefore assumes that the infant has good evolutive potential even if this is not yet fully expressed. This confidence, however, is insufficient for infants at high neurological risk. The CNME attempts to eliminate the significance of transient anomalies by anticipating development.

3. The CNME focuses only on the motor responses that are similar in nature to subsequent motor activity, that is the nonreflex motor activity that the infant will use later in life. The basic hypothesis is as follows: in the liberated state the newborn or young infant demonstrates motor activity like that of an older child that is similar as well to that of the fetus observed in ultrasound examinations [11]. It appears that the same motor activity is present from the prenatal period. Its disappearance during the first weeks seems to be transient and linked to multiple factors, among which the temporary impotence of the neck plays an essential role.

It is important to note, once again, that there is no contradiction between the CNME and the classical neurological examination. The CNME demonstrates the intact and relational motor capacities of high-risk newborns, with the goal of making an early prediction of the absence of major dysfunction of the motor and possibly the cognitive system. The classical neurological examination allows for the identification of transient motor anomalies during the first year and will allow for future correlation with minor handicap at school age.

The CNME allows for an optimistic outlook for high-risk newborns in their first months of life, but this is restricted to predicting the ability to stand and walk unassisted at roughly the normal age. Such information would obviously be helpful to have for all infants, but it is particularly important for infants at high neurological risk of perinatal origin, especially when the classical neurological examination demonstrates anomalies of tone or development in the first weeks of life. In these cases the CNME gives one the ability to look beyond. It is the best way to show the parents what the child will do in the coming months and to help them understand that complete normalization is expected. Their anxiety is replaced by confidence, and the child is integrated into the family without reservation.

When the responses are imperfect they are neither interpreted nor is this observation immediately communicated. The evaluations are repeated until the fourth or fifth month corrected age, with the goal always being the search for normalcy. Physiotherapy is usually prescribed under the pretext of hastening normal motor performance. Regularly repeating the RLA maneuver may result in finally obtaining a positive response. The prognostic significance of the RLA does not change even when elicited after such a delay; it assures the absence of major motor handicap. However, it also plays a therapeutic role. In our experience the stimulation of the neuromuscular pathways of the abduction of each hip plays a favorable role in the bony development of the hip joints when there is central motor dysfunction. This orthopedic prevention may seem superfluous, since there are few infants who have a cerebral motor handicap; yet it has the advantage, in these infants, of eliminating any delay in their specialized therapy [12]. The families of handicapped infants also have permanent psychological support from the neonatal period. Nothing should differentiate the parents of handicapped babies from other parents in their interaction with the medical team. The same discussions should take place between them and the neonatal team without promises and without too early a *pronouncement* of the possibility of an infirmity, which may disturb the relationship of the infant and parents.

References

[1] Grenier A. Révélation d'une expression motrice différente par fixation manuelle de la nuque. In: *Evaluation neurologique du nouveau-né et du nourrisson*, C. Amiel-Tison and A. Grenier (Eds.), pp. 81–102. Masson, Paris, 1980.

[2] Le Métayer M. Contribution à l'étude des schèmes neuromoteurs du nouveau-né et du nourrisson (intérêt dans l'éducation thérapeutique précoce). *Neuropsych. Adol., 11–12*, 587–600, 1981.

[3] Vojta V. *Die cerebralen Bewegungsstörungen im Saüglingsalter. Fruhdiagnose und Fruhtherapie.* F. Enke Verlag, Stuttgart, 1974.

[4] Grenier A. Examen neuromoteur complémentaire. Réaction latérale d'abduction du membre inférieur terminant un enchaînement moteur de l'hémicorps (motricité dirigée). In: *Evaluation neurologique du nouveau-né et du nourrisson*, C. Amiel-Tison and A. Grenier (Eds.), pp. 51–79. Masson, Paris, 1980.

[5] Milani-Comparetti A. The neurophysiologic and clinical implications of the studies on fetal motor behavior. *Semin. Perinatol.*, 5, 2, 183–189, 1981.

[6] Amiel-Tison C. Evolution normale au cours de la 1re année. Repérage des anomalies. Utilisation d'une grille. In: *Evaluation neurologique du nouveau-née et du nourrisson*, C. Amiel-Tison and A. Grenier (Eds.), pp. 10–50. Masson, Paris, 1980.

[7] Grenier A., Vima P., Solomiac J. and Solomiac J. Examen neuromoteur complémentaire chez les nourrissons suspects d'IMC. *Cahiers du Cercle de Documentation et d'Information pour la Rééducation des I.M.C.*, Paris, 65, 1975.

[8] Grenier A. Motricité libérée par fixation manuelle de la nuque au cours des premières semaines de la vie. *Arch. Fr. Pédiatr.*, 38, 557–562, 1981.

[9] Grenier A. A propos de la normalité sensori-motrice néonatale. Son rôle dans le prédépistage. In: *Naissance du cerveau*, pp. 177–182. Nestlé-Guigoz, Monaco, 22–23 April 1982.

[10] Grenier A. La convalescence du nouveau-né à risque. *Ann. Pédiatr.* 32, 41–45, 1985.

[11] Ianniruberto A. and Tajani E. Ultrasonographic study of fetal movements. *Semin. Perinatol.*, 5, 175, 1981.

[12] Grenier A. Diagnostic précoce de l'IMC. Pourquoi faire? *Ann. Pédiatr.*, 7, 509–514, 1982.

5

PROPOSAL FOR AN EVALUATION OF NEUROMOTOR SEQUELAE

The age of 1 year is the usual time to make a prognosis on the motor abilities of a child, even though this initial conclusion may be subject to revision in a few cases. Therefore, the pediatrician who has followed the infant from birth and who has delayed the formulation of a diagnosis of motor handicap can no longer assume the responsibility of following the infant and must send her or him to a specialized team. It is the inevitable time for the pediatrician to make a provisional assessment of the child's abilities with the parents.

FIXED OR NONFIXED MOTOR DYSFUNCTION IN AN INFANT

It is between 4 and 5 months corrected age and the end of the first year that the interpretation of a motor anomaly is the most difficult. The older the infant the harder it is to remain hopeful that it is a transient anomaly and the more likely it is that this anomaly represents a sequela. It is similarly difficult, with disturbed motor function at these ages, to measure the extent of the repercussions there will be on standing and locomotion, on behavior, or on interaction.

These effects may be temporary and reversible, or they may be permanent and progressive. Even in the most favorable cases, however, it is not possible to measure immediately all the consequences on future acquisitions, either motor or nonmotor. It is necessary at this early age to have a basis for interpreting the situation as a whole for the family, in order to begin the best available therapy and to evaluate the extent of damage as much as possible. This is usually based on the motor anomaly that appears to be the most dominant. Generally what

146

is used is a topographical classification (hemiplegia, paraplegia, quadriplegia, etc.), a pathophysiological classification (spastic, athetoid, ataxic,
etc.), and/or a lesional classification defining a pyramidal, extrapyra-
midal, or cerebellar syndrome.

At this early age, though, these classifications—except possibly the
topographical—are not meaningful. The differentiation of syndromes is
not yet possible. The infant may appear to be very hypotonic or very
stiff; such stiffness is too often abusively labeled as a spasticity. The
motor expression of a central lesion in the rapidly developing brain is
as yet unformed, undifferentiated, and poorly defined, thereby escap-
ing the definite classifications used for older children. The impossibility of using pathophysiological or lesional classifications does not present any practical difficulty, since these are not accompanied by
therapeutic indications.

EMPIRICAL BASIS OF THE EVALUATION
OF MOTOR DIFFICULTIES

Tardieu was the first [1] to denounce the lack of utility of a neurological
vocabulary for the young infant; he proposed to replace these classifications by an evaluation of multiple motor and nonmotor factors that
might be used to define and to treat each handicap in a specific way.
This multifactorial approach was an advance in the neurological assessment [2]. At the same time [3, 4], we tried to simplify the approach to
motor difficulties, grouping them within a simple framework with a
dual goal: to simplify the explanations to the family who want to understand, for example, why cerebral damage would lead to orthopedic
treatment of the hips; and second, to simplify the classification of motor problems for the doctor and the physiotherapist.

To do this we divided the necessary elements of normal motor function in a simplistic way. All execution of movement requires a certain
integrity of the CNS, but also requires muscles, bones, and joints in
perfect shape to execute the orders. For the convenience of language
a distinction was made between *problem of neurological command* and
problem in the tools of body function—each indicating different therapy. A third description becomes important as the child grows: *inadequate environment*. The environment in which the infant develops must
sometimes be corrected by therapeutic action.

The term problems of command refers to the disorganization of the
normal means by which automatic and voluntary movements are executed in time and space. These problems involve, for example, ges-

tures that cannot be correctly executed. The regulation, coordination, and distribution of effective muscular contractions may be totally or partially disturbed. Problem of the body tools, on the other hand, refers to a disorder secondary to a cerebral lesion that alters the elementary ability of gesturing [5]. Changes occur in the stretch reflex, in the basic state of the muscles; they are excessively resistant to stretching [2], so that muscular development is disturbed (resulting in overall growth impairment of the affected limb). Problems of the body tools also include secondary alterations that appear with time affecting the muscles, which adapt little by little to a defective position [2], and also the bones, the joints, and particularly the structure of the pelvis, knees, feet and muscles of phonation [6].

From these three components (command, body tools, and environment) an initial functional profile can be formulated around the age of 1 year if there appear to be motor sequelae. It goes without saying that at this early age this functional profile will be based only on standing and locomotion, since the prognosis of walking is the primary interest of the moment. This is therefore only a partial view that does not consider the global effect of the handicap; specifically, it ignores the quality of the movements of the upper extremities, which remain uncertain at this age. Though limited, this evaluation is not necessarily superficial or purely clinical. Standing and locomotion are clearly dominated by the pelvic girdle. In cases of possible impairment there will be repeated x-ray examinations of the hips. The future can be compromised, right from the neonatal period, by negligence or poor interpretation of the growth axes of the neck of the femur and the acetabulum.

FUNCTIONAL PROFILE AT 1 YEAR

We use a simple table (Table 5-1) for the functional profile. On it we can indicate the level of acquisition attained by the infant, the acquisitions not yet present, and the interpretation of the failures as a function of the three components defined above (command, body tools, and environment).

During the first year it is the major functions that are evaluated: head control while prone, and control of sitting and standing (with and without support). Failure at any of these levels can be approached in a subtle way that easily lends itself to a gradation according to the three levels, A, B, and C:

Level A means that the infant maintains the posture in which he is placed by the examiner but cannot assume that posture on his own.

Table 5-1 Functional Gradation for the Evaluation of Failure in Sitting and Standing

| | Gradation of problem | | | |
Motor function	A (maintains only)	B (assumes alone)	C (complete ability)	Interpretation of failure[a]
Seated on a table				
Seated on the edge of a table				
Standing with support				
Standing without support				
Walking				

[a]The interpretation of failure is expressed as a function of the three components: command, body tools, and environment.

Level B indicates a better performance; the infant can assume the posture himself but requires all his attention to do so. The upper extremities are used only for support.

Level C is the highest; the infant assumes the position, leaves it, and reassumes it on his own. He can use all of his attention to gesture without disturbing the position.

For example, the sitting position on a table is at level C at ~8 months of age in a normal baby. If it is absent (level A) or incomplete (level B) at this age, it is necessary to interpret this failure: why is the baby not able to sit unassisted (failure at level B)? The cause may be a profound problem of motor organization or hypertonia of the lower extremities; alternatively, the child may never have learned to sit because of poor environmental stimulation. The normal time of attaining the ability to stand varies from 10 to 18 months. Its absence (level A) or an incomplete ability (level B) cannot be interpreted as pathology until after 18 months of age. Nevertheless it is possible to analyze the reasons for failure. There may be profound problems with motor organization that render the infant incapable of supporting his trunk, or there may be permanent disorders of tone and deformities secondary to that, which make it impossible for him to support his lower extremities. Determining the one factor that predominates among the three (i.e., problems of command, deformity of the body tools, and poor environment) is important in order to make tentative predictions about the near future and to obtain correct therapy.

If there is a *moderate problem of command* the chances are good

Table 5-2   Example of Evaluation of Failure in an Infant Aged 1 Year[a]

Motor function	Gradation of problem			Interpretation of failure[b]
	A (maintains only)	B (assumes alone)	C (complete ability)	
Seated on a table	+	+	0	
Seated on the edge of a table	+	0		
Standing with support	+	0		
Standing without support	0			
Walking				

[a] +, Positive response; 0, failure.
[b] The interpretation of failure is expressed as a function of the three components: command, body tools, and environment.

that, with time and a specialized therapeutic environment, standing and even walking can be reasonably attained, provided the body tools are capable. Corrective and maintenance therapy then become the primary objective; it may be necessary to consider local orthopedic surgery, either curative or preventive. Too often failures of walking are linked years later to subluxation of the hips that occurred because preventive measures were not taken during the first months.

If there is a *major problem of command*, standing will never be possible. Our years of experience have indicated that all attempts at neurological reorganization are doomed to failure; in this situation it is best to work on the body tools in order to prevent major articular deformities, a source of pain and frequent dislocation. The child and the family should be advised of a therapeutic plan that will avoid errors of interpretation and unnecessary treatment.

Let us consider the motor faculties of an infant at age 1 year, such as the one described in Table 5-2. She can sit alone on a table but she cannot use the position to manipulate. Placed at the edge of the table with legs hanging, she uses only her upper extremities for support. She stands with the support of her lower extremities. If her upper extremities are freed by supporting the trunk, they do not move usefully; she puts them in a chandelier position and/or they make disordered movements. To consider helping this infant to sit by a tendinotomy or neurotomy at the level of the adductors will be of no functional benefit. The problem is one of command and not of the tools or the learning environment.

It must also be remembered that in all cases of frank pathological findings the neonatologist must refer the infant for care by a multidisciplinary team like CAMSP (Centre d'Action Médico-Sociale Précoce, specialized multidisciplinary follow-up clinics for high-risk infants used for diagnosis and treatment). If such a team is not available, it is essential to find the most competent specialist and avoid an anonymous referral for reeducation by a physicotherapist outside the medical field [7].

FLUCTUATIONS IN FAILURE AND SUCCESS AS A FUNCTION OF DEVELOPMENT

Aside from the extreme cases, nothing is more difficult with the 1-year-old child than to make a prognosis on the evolution of a handicap, the expression of which changes with ongoing development. A handicap that strongly affects standing, locomotion, and gesturing may almost completely disappear during the second year or even later [8]. Another type, which is in fact fixed, can be seen as becoming more and more incapacitating, mimicking a progressive encephalopathy. This is a fundamental concept: although the lesion itself is stable, its effect may become more profound as the individual develops. Therefore, prolonged surveillance of the body tools becomes indispensable, since new deformities can appear at any time during childhood. It is for this reason that therapy and surveillance are protracted and results at any isolated point in time are difficult to interpret.

For example, the ability to stand during the first year even with poor-quality plantar support does not guarantee that several years later the child will be able to move around other than in a wheelchair. A period of progress can be followed by a phase of deterioration, when standing becomes impossible because the extremities are too stiff, the hips dislocated, and/or the feet deformed. Inversely, a child who at 1 year was unable even to sit may acquire after several years the ability to walk (perhaps with assistance).

In conclusion, analyzing motor problems from the first year in terms of the three aforementioned components gives a practical approach free of all pathophysiological interpretation. It provides a means of communicating with the parents on a practical level, since their observations are the same as ours. They can begin to understand why a surgical procedure on the hip or a tendon would be indicated when the injured organ is the brain, and inversely they will not have unrealistic expectations that such a limited surgical procedure will resolve the overall motor problem.

References

[1] Tardieu G. Infirmité Motrice Cérébrale. *Rev. Neuro-Psychiatr. Infant.*, 1–2, 1, 1968.

[2] Tardieu G. and Tardieu C. "Rétraction," "Hypertonie," "Hypotonie," "Hyperextensibilité," "Hypoextensibilité." Evaluation et indications thérapeutiques. Nécessité d'une évaluation factorielle. *Neuro-Psychiatr. Enf.*, 29, 11–12, 553–567, 1981.

[3] Grenier A. Essai de classification factorielle des troubles moteurs chez les I.M.C. *Kinésithérapie*, 41, 174, 13–20, 1967.

[4] Grenier A. Contribution au traitement des troubles de l'organisation motrice chez l'I.M.C. *Cahier du Cercle de Documentation et d'Information pour la Rééducation des I.M.C.*, 34, 5–54, 1967.

[5] Tardieu G. and Tabary J. C. Considération sur l'athétose de l'enfant. *Arch. Fr. Pédiatr.*, 22, 289–316, 1965.

[6] Tardieu G. and Chevrie-Muller C. Evaluation factorielle, indications et contreindications thérapeutiques dans les troubles du langage et de la déglutition chez l'I.M.C. *Neuro-Psychiatr. Enf.*, 29, 11–12, 613–623, 1981.

[7] Truscelli D. Infirmité motrice centrale. Bilan et prise en charge. *Rev. Pédiatr.*, 20, 1, 35–42, 1984.

[8] Ellenberg J. H. and Nelson K. B. Children who "outgrew" cerebral palsy. *Pediatrics*, 69, 529–536, 1982.

6

SIGNIFICANCE OF TRANSIENT NEUROMOTOR ANOMALIES AND THEIR CORRELATION WITH DIFFICULTIES AT SCHOOL AGE

GOALS IN THE CORRELATION BETWEEN THE FIRST YEAR AND SCHOOL AGE

It would be nice to believe that cerebral plasticity in the newborn is such that initial neurological signs most often disappear, and no trace of perinatal asphyxia remains. The tendency for motor signs to disappear completely in the course of rapid maturation during the first year lends hope to the above view. When at age 7 years the child begins to exhibit minor neurological signs and behavior problems, resulting in the diagnosis of MBD, the motor symptomatology of the first year is most often forgotten, if it was recognized at all.

In the preface of her book on MBD, Rapin [1] summarizes this point of view: "Plasticity, the capacity for reorganization after an injury, was assumed until fairly recently to be so great in the immature brain that full behavioral recovery was thought to be the rule in young children unless damage was extensive. We have come to appreciate that plasticity is limited, and that recovery without discernible deficit is in fact uncommon."

It is in this perspective that a grid for the neuromotor examination in the first year was proposed in an attempt to link these perinatal events and subsequent moderate deficits in a logical manner. We feel this is a realistic point of view that allows for more appropriate guidance for the group of infants who will have a permanent neuromotor or psychic deficit. It is possible that the eventual handicap will not be detectable using our examination techniques; still, if a handicap is present, why ignore it or deny its links to perinatal cellular damage?

153

We agree with Rapin that cerebral plasticity was probably overestimated without sufficient proof and that cerebral sequelae of perinatal origin are extremely polymorphic. The spectrum of deficits goes from mild to severe.

Accepting the above facts does not contradict the need for a program of early intervention at all stages of development: motor activity, language, and finally adaptation to school. All attempts at helping the parents to accept the child and to strengthen the familial bond are useful; they are the essential continuation of early interaction as stressed by Brazelton [2]. The usefulness of this overall therapeutic approach is intuitively obvious even if it is impossible to demonstrate. The child with a handicap, minor or major, is a child who risks parental rejection at any time. Those who work with abused children know this and consider this a useful approach [3]; why look for other arguments?

Finally, obstetricians cannot wait for school age to evaluate the results of their decisions or techniques, but they can review the statistical risk of moderate anomalies during the first year. This feedback is another important reason for the identification of transient motor signs during the first year.

Current data and our personal results are here analyzed. We discuss the transient nature of neuromotor anomalies as well as the methodology of preschool evaluation and the importance of this correlation in prevention and guidance.

CURRENT DATA

In 1972 Drillien described a group of anomalies of tone seen in a group of LBW infants; these were transient anomalies followed until motor normalization occurred at 18 months [4]. These children were followed until school age and were compared to children of similar birth weight without anomalies during the first year as well as to a control group of full-term newborns of normal weight [5, 6]. These children (with the exception of six who had cerebral motor handicaps) were all tested between ages 6 and 8 by a battery of tests: IQ, scholastic results, motor function, and perceptual function. A final overall handicap score was calculated from 0 to 3: the children who scored 0 or 1 had good adjustment to school, those with a score of 2 had minor problems, and those with a score of 3 had significant problems. The controls were matched according to socioeconomic group. The results were as follows: there was no significant differences between the LBW infants without anomalies and the control group; however, among the LBW infants with transient motor difficulties, 23% had considerable difficul-

Table 6-1 Extent of Handicap as Expressed by a Total Score, Determined by a Battery of Tests between 6 and 8 Years[a]

Final handicap score	Neurological abnormalities (%)	No neurological abnormalities (%)	Controls (%)
0	31	55	68
1	33	28	16
2	13	8	12
3	23	9	4
Number of cases	100	131	111

Source: Reproduced with permission from C. M. Drillien, in *Major mental handicap*, Ciba Foundation Symposium, no. 59. Elsevier, New York, 1978.

[a] Subjects included LBW infants who experienced motor anomalies during the first year of life, LBW infants with no motor anomalies during the first year of life, and a control group.

ties between 6 and 8 years (score of 3), as opposed to 9% in the LBW group without anomalies and 4% in the control group (Table 6-1). These numbers, published in 1978 and then in 1980, were the first to show the subsequent significance of having had transient motor signs in the first year. These data are for very small prematures who because of the time of their birth were treated by less sophisticated methods than currently available in intensive care. The neurological signs observed during the first year were described by the term "dystonic syndrome," which we do not use, but the group of signs remains classic: troubles of tone and hyperexcitability. The long-term results preliminarily reported by Drillien in 1978 during a Ciba symposium on transient neuromotor anomalies observed in full-term newborns showed that the trail was reliable and that the same continuity of deficits would probably be seen in full-term infants as had been seen in prematures. These results also showed that in children who had motor problems identified during their first year, MBD was not always found to be present at school age; indeed, 64% of Drillien's affected group had no identifiable school problems (31% scored 0 and 33% scored 1). The data demonstrated that too many infants were initially included in the group at risk, and therefore early individual prognosis was unwise. However, the data also demonstrated that about one-quarter of the infants who were identified at risk during their first year but were considered to have normalized by age 1 year, would subsequently be part of the group with true cerebral deficits at school age.

Included in the Ciba symposium were other groups that have reported similar results for neuromotor signs seen in the first year, showing future risk associated with these transient signs [7, 8].

In recent years several studies, often using large numbers of children, have shown similar results for the evolution of neuromotor anomalies observed during the first year. They may persist (usually diminished), change their expression, or disappear.

The work of Rubin and Balow [9] used a cohort of 1319 children who were part of the Collaborative North American Project of Perinatal Research. During this longitudinal prospective study three neurological examinations were done during the first year, which allowed the classification of these infants in three groups: normal, suspect and abnormal. These children were followed until age 12 years with psychomotor tests, batteries of tests of fine motor function, and scholastic results. Socioeconomic class and birth weight were statistically controlled. The analysis of performance at a later age for the three initial groups showed a strong correlation between neuromotor anomaly in the first year (even transient) and risk at school age. Approximately 29% of the children in the "abnormal" group in the first year had IQs <70 at age 4 years, as opposed to 1.9% in the "suspect" group and 1% in the "normal" group. Analysis of these results shows that the association is not strong enough to justify an individual prediction, but it confirms the value of indicating the risk of anomalies observed during the first year.

The work of Nelson and Ellenberg [10] had similar results and brought attention to the overdiagnosis of cerebral palsy during the first year, since motor anomalies observed were transient in 118 of the 229 children who were evaluated during their first year as being handicapped. However, among these 118 children whose motor difficulties disappeared, it was found that 13% of the white children and 25% of the black children had an IQ <70 at age 7 years. It was also found that this group had an elevated incidence of seizure with fever, language difficulties, and behavioral problems.

Another prospective study, that of Ellison *et al.* [11], confirmed this result: 237 children were followed after discharge from the intensive care unit and had neuromotor examinations at 6 and 15 months corrected age. At age 4 years they were tested by the McCarthy and a battery of tests for fine motor and sensorimotor coordination. The results showed a correlation between motor coordination and the presence of a motor dysfunction during the first year ($P < 0.01$).

PERSONAL RESULTS

We proposed a strong correlation between transient neuromotor anomalies and problems at school age from our initial publication of a de-

Table 6-2 Classification at 1 Year of Age according to Neuromotor Evaluation of 36 Infants Regularly Followed since Birth

Study within the first year	Number of cases	
Lost to follow-up within the first year	9	
Normal all during the first year	5	
Transient abnormalities within the first year	29	36
Cerebral palsy	2	
Total number	45	

scription of the neuromotor anomalies of the first year in 1976 [12], and then again with our original results for full-term newborns following perinatal asphyxia [13]. Our recent results [14] confirmed these findings by showing that deviations from normal motor development in the first year act as a thread that leads to other anomalies that appear in subsequent years. Thus these early deviations are an indication for prolonged surveillance.

Fifteen children studied at school age represented half of the cohort of a prospective study begun in the neonatal period in 1975 at the Port-Royal Maternity Hospital in Paris; 45 children had long-term surveillance as a result of the presence of neurological anomalies at the end of the first week of life, excluding cases of malformation or infection. Of 36 infants followed through the first year, 29 had transient anomalies (Table 6-2) and were considered normal at age 1 year (16 normalized between 1 and 3 months and 13 normalized between 4 and 12 months). These children then returned one or two times a year until the examination done between 5 and 6 years. Fifteen children of the cohort group born in the same year (1975), at Port-Royal Maternity Hospital, came for this examination, as did 15 controls who were chosen on the basis of an absence of any neurological signs during the first week of life. The examination at 5 to 6 years involved a classical neurological evaluation, including, in particular, evaluation for dyspraxias of the mouth and fingers. Static and dynamic equilibrium was tested. Cortical function was evaluated by different tests of ideomotor adaptation evaluating precision and rapidity of gestures. As part of the neurological examination, a psychologist administered the Terman–Merrill test and did a behavioral evaluation during the test. The neuropediatrician also evaluated behavior during his examination, and the parents

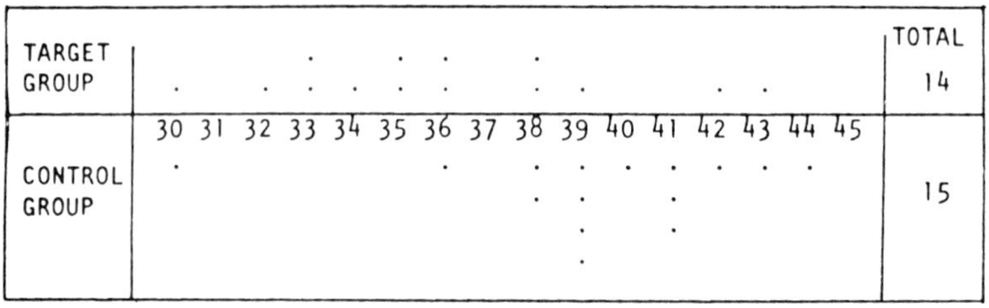

TARGET GROUP					.	.	.		.							TOTAL 14
	.		.	.	.	.		.		.	.			.	.	
	30	31	32	33	34	35	36	37	38	39	40	41	42	43	44	45
CONTROL GROUP	.					.			.		.	.	.	.	.	.	15
									.		.		.			
									.							

Fig. 6-1 Global performance score for the two groups.

filled out a questionnaire on behavior at home. These tests were administered in a blind fashion for all 30 infants.

The classical neurological examination results were classified as either normal or abnormal (i.e., an anomaly was noted). The other tests were scored on a basis of 0 to 3 (0 represented the absence of response, 1 and 2 an intermediate response, and 3 the optimal response). All the children cooperated without problem for the whole evaluation, which involved two sessions of 30 to 40 minutes during one half-day. The main results can be summarized as follows.

For the *neuromotor tests* the scores were added for a maximum score of 45; a score <36 was considered abnormal, as seen in seven subjects and one control (Fig. 6-1).

In the *classical neurological examination*, five subjects were found to have abnormalities in praxic function and one of them was subsequently found to have a seizure disorder. Two controls also failed the praxis tests (Table 6-3).

The results of psychomotor testing (Terman–Merrill) are expressed in Fig. 6-2 using global IQ only in the two groups: in the control group IQ is always >100 and well clustered; the results are widely dispersed in the affected group, and in three cases IQ is ≤85.

For a final classification three categories were defined according to

Table 6-3 Dyspraxic Movements of the Tongue and/or Fingers in the Classical Neurological Examination

	Normal neurological examination	Dyspraxia	Total
Subjects	10	5	15
Controls	13	2	15

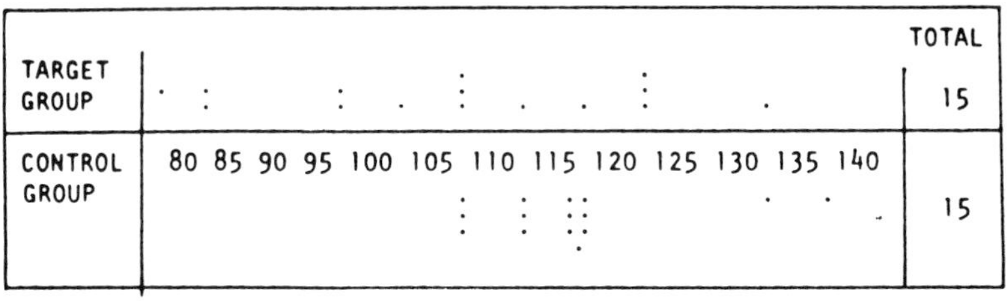

		TOTAL
TARGET GROUP	· : : · : · · : ·	15
CONTROL GROUP	80 85 90 95 100 105 110 115 120 125 130 135 140 : : :: · · .	15

Fig. 6-2   Development quotient for the two groups.

the results obtained in the three objective parts of the evaluation: the neurological examination, the tests of motor performance, and the IQ.

Abnormal: Anomalies existed in two of the three components of the evaluation.
Intermediate: Anomalies existed in one of the components.
Normal: All performances were satisfactory.

The results as expressed in Table 6-4 are as follows: 13 of the 15 controls were normal; 5 of the 15 subjects were normal, 4 were abnormal; 6 children were in the intermediate group and required subsequent evaluation. In spite of the small size of the cohort, the results are significant at $p < 0.005$.

SENSITIVITY OF THE METHOD OF CLINICAL EVALUATION BETWEEN 5 AND 6 YEARS

The choice of methods of evaluation at preschool age is difficult; there is no satisfactory standardization to allow for the interpretation of a response as optimal at a given age, and even the choice of tests must be defined. The group of tests used must not be too sophisticated nor too complicated to be applicable and reproducible. We found our choices

Table 6-4   Classification at Age 5–6 Years in Three Categories Based on Neurological Exam, Global Performance Score, and IQ Evaluation

Number of cases	Categories at 5–6 years		
	Abnormal	Intermediate	Normal
Target group 15 children	4	6	5
Control group 15 children	1	1	13

satisfactory, since they allowed us to evaluate cerebral function and behavior in an exhaustive way, and since they uncovered problems in 2 of 15 controls, a reasonable percentage of 13% for a population considered normal at 5 to 6 years of age. It can therefore be concluded that the borderline was well positioned between the presence and absence of problems and that this method did not lose itself in the search for problems that are too minor to be of interest. At the same time the method was sensitive enough to demonstrate deficits that had escaped notice by parents and teachers.

Current imaging techniques are not sensitive enough to provide useful information on the morphological basis of minor deficits. This issue has not been addressed in our work nor in any of the studies cited, since in the years of birth of the children in these studies the CT scan was used only in cases of severe neonatal disorder and ultrasound did not yet exist. Later CT scan done at the time when MBD becomes evident is also very deceptive. We can give only one example, the case of the most severely handicapped child of the cohort group. This was a little girl who had a seizure disorder from the age of 18 months, was clearly dyspraxic, and had an IQ of 83. The signs of cerebral damage observed in the neonatal period were clearly associated with acute distress in the beginning of labor in a fetus at 42 weeks' gestation; signs of CNS depression were observed during the first weeks, and two isolated seizures were observed during the first days of life. Results of the CT scan done at 5 years for the seizure disorder and at the same time as the preschool clinical evaluation were normal.

At the present time it is the clinical evaluation that provides most information, but other methods are most likely being developed that will allow fine correlation between the clinical evaluation of a deficit and the morphological anomaly.

WHY ARE CERTAIN NEUROMOTOR ANOMALIES TRANSIENT, AND ARE THEY?

This question has long preoccupied many workers in the field, and the recent accumulation of data has only shown the diversity of possibilities and therefore the impossibility of arriving at a simple and unequivocal answer.

Sometimes the demands are lost during the second year rather than the anomalies disappearing. During the first year it is the precision of maturative events in the motor domain that allows for the establish-

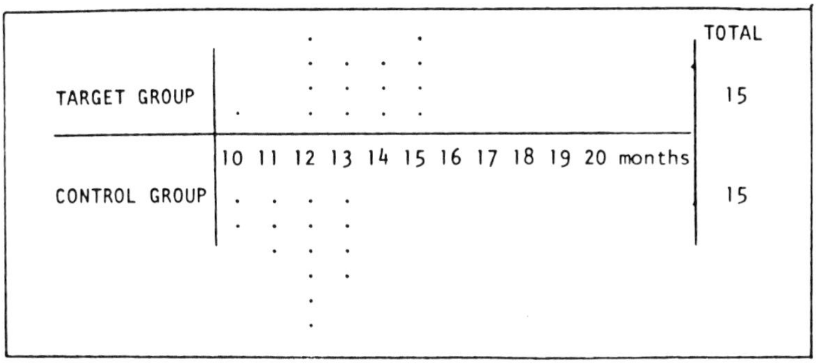

Fig. 6-3   Age of independent walking in the two groups.

ment of the limits of normal development and therefore deviations from normal. But when the pace of development slows during the second year the limits of normalcy lose their precision. The example of the *age of walking* is particularly clear: for a long time the limit between acquiring walking at a normal and abnormal age has been fixed empirically at 18 months; this definition is wise, since familial or individual variations are great and no prediction of function should be based on the few months difference of acquiring this ability between 1 and 1½ years of age. If we look at the age of walking in our series (Fig. 6-3), the 15 children with transient motor anomalies walked before 18 months; that is, we observed no delay in walking in the classical use of the term. However, they walked significantly later than the controls: all of the controls walked by 13 months, whereas only 8 subjects walked at this age, a significant difference at $p < 0.01$. A similar observation was reported by Cockburn [7] in observing the ability to walk five steps unassisted at age 1 year: only 20% of his group of premature infants was able to do this, as opposed to 50% of the controls. Very recently, results with the same conclusion were reported at the International Congress of Pediatrics [15] on a group of 20 children in whom the age of walking was the only early marker of motor difficulties. Thus, using the simple example of walking, it is easy to show that the "transient" character of motor difficulties is in fact imprecise. Motor problems are not transient, they continue; it is the definition that becomes inaccurate and unsatisfactory. When these children grow it is not surprising for them to score below normal on tests of motor performance at 5 years using simple tests such as walking along a straight line, hopping on one foot, maintaining balance, tiptoeing. However, such subtle deficits often escape the attention of the family and school.

It is likely that similar results will be seen for the more complex evaluation of fine motor function. If efforts are directed toward meticulously observing sensorimotor coordination at the ages of 2, 3, and 4 years (the most difficult ages for cooperation) with precise methodology such as that used by Denckla [16], Ellison [11], and many others, it becomes quite clear that the "silent period" of preschool age does not really exist. There is a methodological problem in the evaluation rather than a missing link.

Even if it is recognized that for each function a continuity exists and that the difficulty comes essentially from our poor observation of minor deficits, it is still true that motor function seems to improve as maturation progresses. The observations of Knobloch and Pasamanick [17] allowed them to suggest that after the age of 1 year a more precise motor function appears, giving the child control over minor deficits; Solomons *et al.* [18] made similar observations.

In our clinical observations during the first year, it was striking to notice the *abrupt nature* of motor "normalization," which could often be interpreted as a phenomenon linked to maturation. The following typical situation in a high-risk infant is a good example:

The association of hyperexcitability and a deficit of tone in the upper part of the body is observed during the first months; suddenly, in a matter of days the situation changes at the time head control is finally acquired. It is thought that the initial insult was so modest as to disturb only the most recently acquired function transiently (tonus of flexors of the head and upper extremities). Head control is acquired at a normal or slightly delayed age, and once this stage is reached, all signs of motor dysfunction that were "subcortical" disappear completely. It is rare for an infant who had early normalization to have future deficits. One can imagine that it is the progressive functional "wiring" of the brain during maturation that results in the eradication of the effects of minor dysfunction—if they do not affect future acquisitions.

In order for a deficit to be evident, function must be established. This obvious statement explains the slowness with which cognitive deficits are uncovered in the course of development and therefore the way the psychologists are fooled in their detection of moderate deficits before the age of 2 years (see Chapter 7).

However, it is sometimes possible to bypass the difficulty and anticipate future function. The best example of this is in the evaluation of hand–eye coordination before it is permanently acquired when the examiner temporarily provides head control. This is an anticipation that likely has prognostic value for the function evaluated (see Chapter 4).

IMPORTANCE OF THE CONTINUING NEUROMOTOR THREAD FOR PREVENTION

The available data in the literature and our personal experience have shown the correlation that exists between transient neuromotor anomalies in the first year and MBD at school age. The existence of this correlation, even if imperfect, encourages the careful observation of transient signs all throughout the first year. This observation has two objectives:

1. There is *an individual objective* for each of the children, since establishing the thread means foreseeing possible moderate deficits in the future, which also means prolonged guidance. Certainly complete normalization will be seen in about half of the cases, and it is important to enhance the normalization by avoiding unjustified anxiety on the part of the family. In the other cases, early recognition of the problem can make it possible for the child to be helped—possibly by direct action, and always by helping the family recognize the "difference" in their child. If the body tools are not perfect, special assistance will be required all throughout school and until the time comes for the individual to choose a profession.

2. A Public Health objective also exists, in the form of evaluating the current techniques of intensive care, both neonatal and obstetrical. The common objective of all perinatal care, whether preventive or therapeutic, is to have a survivor with an intact brain. Therefore, it is important to furnish results that are both rapid and precise—that is, not to be satisfied with merely knowing the number of children with profound sequelae at the end of the first year of life. The best information is provided by the neuromotor marker, because it has statistical significance for the risk of minor cerebral handicap at school age.

References

[1] Rapin I. *Children with brain dysfunction*. Raven Press, New York, 1982.
[2] Brazelton T. B. Early intervention, what does it mean? In: *Therapy and research in behavioral pediatrics*, vol. 1, H. E. Fitzgerald, B. M. Lester and M. Yogman, (Eds.), pp. 1–33, Plenum Publications, New York, 1982.

[3] Bax M. Abuse and cerebral palsy. *Dev. Med. Child Neurol.*, 25, 141–142, 1983.

[4] Drillien C. M. Abnormal neurologic signs in the first year of life in low birth weight infants. Possible prognostic significance. *Dev. Med. Child Neurol.*, 14, 575, 1972.

[5] Drillien C. M. Discussion. In: *Major mental handicap*, Ciba Foundation Symposium, no. 59, p. 120. Elsevier, Amsterdam, 1978.

[6] Drillien C. M., Thomson A. J. M. and Burgoyne K. Low birth weight children at early school age: a longitudinal study. *Dev. Med. Child Neurol.*, 22, 26–47, 1980.

[7] Cockburn F. Discussion. In: *Major mental handicap*, Ciba Foundation Symposium, no. 59, p. 121. Elsevier, Amsterdam, 1978.

[8] Micheli J. L. Discussion. In: *Major mental handicap*, Ciba Foundation Symposium, no. 59, p. 123. Elsevier, Amsterdam, 1978.

[9] Rubin R. A. and Balow B. Infant neurological abnormalities as indicators of cognitive impairment. *Dev. Med. Child Neurol.*, 22, 336–343, 1980.

[10] Nelson K. B. and Ellenberg J. H. Children who "outgrew" cerebral palsy. *Pediatrics*, 69, 529–536, 1982.

[11] Ellison P. H., Prasse D. P., Siewart J. and Browning C. A. Correlations of neurologic assessment in infancy with fine motor, gross motor, and intellectual assessment at four years in a neonatal intensive care unit population. In: *Intensive care in the newborn, IV*, L. Stern, H. Bard and B. Friis-Hansen (Eds.), pp. 241–246. Masson, New York, 1983.

[12] Amiel-Tison C. A method for neurologic evaluation within the first year of life. *Curr. Prob. Pediatr.*, 7, 5, 1976.

[13] Amiel-Tison C. A method for neurological evaluation within the first year of life: experience with full term newborn infants with birth injury. In: *Major mental handicap*, Ciba Foundation Symposium no. 59, pp. 107–126. Elsevier, Amsterdam, 1978.

[14] Amiel-Tison C., Dube R., Garel M. and Jequier J. C. Outcome at age five years of full-term infant with transient neurologic abnormalities in the first year of life. In: *Intensive care in the newborn, IV*, L. Stern, H. Bard and B. Friis-Hansen (Eds.), pp. 247–258. Masson, New York, 1983.

[15] Pe Benito R., Ferretti C. and Fisch C. B. Residual neurological disabilities in children with "resolved" cerebral palsy. *17th International Congress of Pediatrics Abstracts*, 2, p. 83, Manila, 1983.

[16] Denckla M. B. Development of motor co-ordination in normal children. *Dev. Med. Child Neurol.*, 16, 729–741, 1974.

[17] Knobloch H. and Pasamanick B. *Gesell and Armatruda's development diagnosis*, 3rd ed. Harper & Row, New York, 1974.

[18] Solomons G., Holden R. H. and Denhoff E. The changing picture of cerebral dysfunction in early childhood. *Pediatrics*, 63, 113–120, 1963.

7

THE PLACE OF
DEVELOPMENTAL SCALES
AND SENSORY EVALUATION

Discussion of developmental scales and sensory evaluation is deliberately placed at the end of this book, which has attempted to describe the neuromotor examination of the young infant in a personal way, stressing its priorities. The location of this discussion also reflects our feelings of being "accomplices after the fact." We want to take advantage of these important data that were collected independently by our colleagues to evaluate a child as completely as possible.

For a long time the psychomotor developmental scales have been the major tool in the follow-up of infants at risk, and this continues to be the case—perhaps too frequently. In fact the numbers obtained by developmental quotient (DQ) tests allow for easy categorization; it was comfortable for the neurologists to accept this, and they maintained a "hands-off" attitude. Now, the presence of psychologists and their methods of evaluation are recognized as necessary in a follow-up clinic, but this represents only one part of the evaluation.

Along the same lines, sensorial evaluation has taken a place of greater importance with the improvement of techniques. Much recent work has emphasized the risks of visual and auditory deficits for which signs and symptoms are not very specific. A sensorial handicap, as yet unrecognized, will result in a low IQ, but for reasons other than cognitive or neuromotor problems. A true polydisciplinary evaluation is therefore indispensable if the risks are to be understood and their consequences minimized.

The Developmental Scales

HISTORY

The name Arnold Gesell has remained strongly linked to the field of normal psychomotor development. His studies on the development of infants were done at Yale University in the 1920s [1]; standardization and the materials used for testing became widespread in the 1940s [2]. Then the whole of Gesell's works were put into a book on the first 5 years of life in the form of a "guide to the study of the preschool child" [3]. In effect, his work on the first year of life led Gesell to continue his study until school age and to show the "organic continuity" that links these 5 years, stating "that identical principles of growth and of guidance apply to infant, toddler, run about and school beginner." This extraordinary work on the child from birth to 5 years has been generally used by those who followed Gesell, and his methods have remained the major influence on techniques to measure psychomotor development.

DESCRIPTION OF THE MOST USEFUL TESTS

The functional level of a child includes quantifiable components such as intellectual ability, motor skill, language, the degree of complexity of perceptions, and affect. This is an inventory of development in which each element can be noted by its presence or absence. In this way it is possible to define a developmental age. The chronological age of the child allows the comparison of his or her level of development with the functional capacities of a group of normal children of the same age, with environmental and genetic factors considered to be average for the population as a whole.

Contemporary with Gesell's work, Nancy Bayley began the California study known as the Berkeley Growth Study; its goal was to follow a sample of children through their lives, studying their individual development with great depth in all medical, psychological, and social aspects. This study continued for 36 years. The mental and motor developmental scales of Bayley were standardized on 1400 children in the 1960s [4]. It is in this form that they are still largely used in the United States. Later, Bayley opened the field of research on prediction of future performance based on observations made during the first years, on the role of the environment, and on the harmonious chain reaction in normal development [5].

Other scales, also inspired by the work of Gesell, are used just as commonly. Among them are that of Griffiths in Great Britain [6] and that of Brunet and Lezine [7] in France. The level of psychomotor development and its evolution are analyzed in four areas: postural development, oculomotor coordination, language, and sociability.

In spite of their similarities, differences exist in each of these developmental scales, for example, the manner of expressing results and the population of children on whom it was initially tested. Each of them describes the responses for specific tasks of increasing difficulty and observations of spontaneous behavior. Some of the scales use information from observations made by the mother; others only use that which is observed in the course of the psychologist's evaluation. The observations are organized systematically in the areas of motor development, adaptive ability, sociability, and communication. The final score is variable: a "mental" score and a "motor" score in the Bayley; an overall score and an individual score for each of the five sections in the Griffiths and the Brunet–Lezine.

Comparing these different scales is difficult because each uses arbitrary cutoffs, different definitions, and different conditions of observation; also, each was standardized on populations hardly comparable. The experience of Ramsay and Fitzhardinge [8] expresses this difficulty very well: the tests of Bayley and Griffiths were given to 50 children at age 1 year; they were administered blind by the same psychologist during the same consultation. The results showed a difference of 10 to 15 points in the score obtained in the two tests, that of Griffiths usually being higher than that of Bayley to a statistically significant degree. This study showed that the results of these two tests are not interchangeable for multiple reasons, among them the separation of the various tests and the socioeconomic level of the normal sample. The results of this work illuminate the need for caution in interpreting the results of these scales and indicate the need for further comparisons of this kind. We can also dream that there will be a unanimous choice of only one of these tests that would eliminate the problem of comparisons. It would also be useful to have a new standardization done on the population of children born in the 1980s.

Aside from the technical aspect of standardization and the problems of comparison, however, the most thorny problem is theoretical [9, 10]. All the existing tests reflect the traditional hypotheses on the development of intelligence. However, for the first years of life the notion of intellectual quotient (IQ) has been replaced by that of developmental quotient (DQ), a concept that allows for the measurement of progress in early childhood. It is hoped that the DQ measured in the beginning stages of development will allow for the prediction of subsequent IQ and the final level of intelligence and competence of an individual. However, the hypothesis that DQ and IQ are static has not been verified, nor has the hypothesis of a predetermined rate of development been established. Even the basis of these tests—that is, the choice of items—has been recently questioned.

It is not possible to continue the theoretical debate on development here, but it is important to note that these tests—such as they are—represent an excellent tool for follow-up and surveillance of high-risk newborns. Certainly classical psychology, although imperfect, along with the neurological examination, has provided the most current results available in the literature. The application of these methods of the LBW newborn as in full-term newborns with abnormality has brought important data to light over the years since the mid-1970s.

NECESSITY OF "CORRECTING" AGE

Development in the first year is completely dependent on the maturation of the nervous system.

Motor development in particular is so rapid and so precise (as represented in Figure 7-1, an example by Bower [11]), that it would not be reasonable to calculate the score based on anything but corrected age.

It would therefore appear to be essential to "correct" the age of the child by subtracting the weeks or months he was premature and using corrected age instead of real age. A demonstration of this has been furnished by Parmelee and Schulte [12], who used the Gesell test on full-term newborns, premature newborns, and hypotrophic newborns in a double-blind study. The results showed that Gesell's tests were dependent on the duration of gestation and that it is indeed necessary to make the correction for age. By making this correction all newborns can be compared, no matter what their conceptional age.

PREDICTIVE VALUE OF THE DEVELOPMENTAL QUOTIENT

The DQ rarely has predictive value before 2 years of age in moderate handicaps. The anxiety of prediction is not new; it is as old as the existence of centers for neonatal intensive care. However, two recent studies have very precisely indicated the answers given by the use of psychomotor tests for the population of newborns at very high risk.

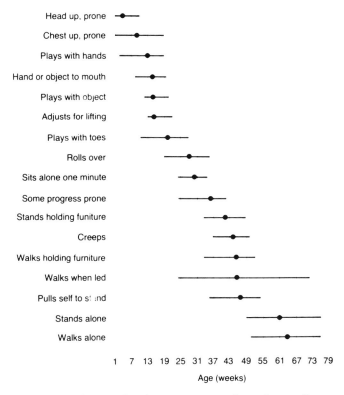

Fig. 7-1 Schedule of motor development up to independent walking. (From Bower T. G. R. *A primer of infant development.* Freeman & Co., San Francisco, 1977, with permission.)

Hunt's results [13]

At the University of California, San Francisco, this study was done on a group of 61 infants weighing 1500 g, born and cared for in the hospital between 1965 and 1972. For the first 2 years researchers used either the Cattell Test of Infant Development or the Bayley Scales for Infant Development at 6 months, and at 1 and 2 years. The Stanford–Binet test was given at 3, 4, 5, and 6 years. Corrected age was used until 2 years. The distribution of scores obtained by these different tests is represented in Figure 7-2. The following observations may be made:

• The children with DQ <70 at 6 months and 1 year always had problems subsequently; therefore, severe abnormality was identified in the first year.

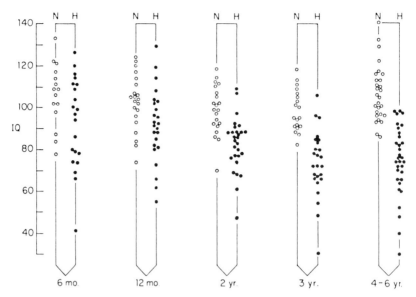

Fig. 7-2 ○ Children with normal test results at 4 to 6 years; ● handicapped children at 4 to 6 years. Distribution of mental test scores for a group of children "at risk," tested from infancy and classified at 4 to 6 years. Comparisons at interval from infancy between the groups that were labeled normal (N) or handicapped (H) at 4 to 6 years. The distinction between these groups is not apparent until after age 2 years.
(From Hunt J. V. Longitudinal research: a method for studying the intellectual development of high-risk preterm infants. In: *Infants born at risk: behavior and development*, T. M. Field, A. M. Sostek, S. Goldberg and H. H. Shuman (Eds.), pp. 443–460. Spectrum Publications, London, 1979, with permission.)

- However, among the infants with DQ >70 at 6 months and 1 year, the tests did not allow for the differentiation of the two populations (normal or moderately handicapped) that become distinct during the second year of life.
- At 2 years, however, a clear separation of the two populations took place: most children who would be normal at 4 to 6 years had a DQ >90, whereas most of those who would be handicapped scored <90, with a few individual exceptions.

The conclusion of this longitudinal study shows the prognostic value of the DQ at 2 years. The prediction is not perfect; it cannot be used for an individual, but it is statistically satisfying.

A DQ <90 at 2 years is a sufficient indication to undertake guidance. The tests allow the examiner to select the children with potential disorders and to suggest the possibility of brain damage, even in the absence of developmental problems in the first year.

Fitzhardinge's results [14]

A prospective study was done at the Toronto Hospital for Sick Children on 133 newborns who weighed 1500 g at birth. A neurological examination was done at 1, 2, and 6 years. The Bayley scales were applied every 6 months during the first 2 years, and a Wechsler scale was performed at 6 years. The diagnosis was made the first year for children who had a major neurological deficit (hydrocephalus and/or cerebral motor disability); the degree of handicap remained constant until 6 years. There was a positive correlation between the Bayley score at all ages and the Wechsler score at 6 years. However, the correlation was only highly significant from 18 to 24 months. At 2 years it was possible to predict the Wechsler score as above or below 85 in 80% of the cases.

In conclusion, major neurological handicap or intellectual deficit or a combination of the two can be predicted at age 2 years with satisfactory precision. However, minor or moderate handicap or intellectual deficit cannot be satisfactorily predicted at this age. Great caution is necessary in making predictions for individual cases.

NECESSITY OF TESTING OTHER FUNCTIONS

The DQ alone does not suffice as a predictor of scholastic difficulties. This was very well shown by Hunt *et al.* [15] by the analysis of learning problems in a group of newborns weighing <1500 g. The final analysis of results includes not only the DQ measured at 4 years by the Stanford–Binet, for which the results are expressed in three levels (pathological, limited, and normal), but also a gradation of problems of comprehension of language and capacity of visuomotor coordination. The overall problems are classified as either frank handicap or moderate difficulty with the possibility of future improvement. The addition of the children with a DQ ≤84 and the children with frank handicap in language comprehension and coordination resulted in a total of 45% at 4 years. On the other hand, the children with a normal DQ and with no overt deficit in comprehension and fine motor activity represented 55% of the population at age 4 years. This anticipation of problems that may lead to a learning disability is evidently of practical interest, so that the best assistance can be offered to these children at the most useful time.

Theoretically, it would be interesting to show the connection of unfavorable perinatal conditions and this group of neurological troubles. Actually, the frequency with which these troubles are observed in the group of VLBW newborns is more than twice the highest estimations for the general population; in addition, the frequency of these learning disabilities is greater than that observed for the siblings of these children.

It is this link of cause and effect that we have tried to demonstrate and foresee in the analysis of transient neuromotor problems of the first year (see Chapter 6). This is what Drillien has shown as well [16], in her analysis of the school performance of a group of premature infants who had transient neuromotor anomalies compared to a group of premature infants having normal motor development.

In conclusion, this brief analysis of method and of results makes us recognize two areas of failure in the predictive value of the DQ of the first years: the impossibility of reassuring the parents before age 2 years and the lack of precision regarding the specific nature of subsequent problems. The developmental scales and the contact established between parents and psychologists during these evaluations are, however, indispensable. The scores on subtests, the dispersed nature of the acquisitions in the child, and the quality of parent–child interaction are often more significant than the overall raw score on the DQ.

The Detection of Sensorial Deficits

The frequency of visual or auditory handicaps in a population of newborns at risk is a widely disputed point. This diversity of opinion is a good example of how something is only found when it is sought. The prognosis of strabismus or amblyopia is known to depend on early treatment, therefore depending on detection during the first year. The development of language depends on correct hearing, and too many children at risk are considered mentally deficient because of undiagnosed deafness.

VISION

The detection of visual problems is a preoccupation in the population at risk made up of mainly LBW children. The number of functional or organic anomalies encountered justifies a regular surveillance with complete examinations oriented toward detecting the most frequent anomalies. The lower the birth weight the more frequently anoxic accidents were likely to occur and the more careful should be the ophthalmological follow-up. In fact, a careful ophthalmological examination should take place during the first year on all "risk" newborns. Severe retinopathy of prematurity, linked to hyperoxygenation, will not be discussed in detail here, since it would be identified while the infant is still hospitalized in the intensive care unit and would already be the subject of careful observation aimed at preventing retinal detachment. The group of problems caused by this complication in the VLBW newborn is the subject of a recent book [17]. All is not yet known about pathogenesis, and in spite of the great efforts to administer oxygen with precision to small premature infants, blindness remains a complication that has not completely disappeared [18]. Similarly, an absence of fixing regard, and nystagmus are clear signs that must indicate immediate examination by a specialist; in such a case it is not a question of detection but of elementary clinical diagnosis.

By contrast, we are more concerned here with the minor complications that are not evident during the first year, but which if detected early can benefit from curative or preventive treatment.

Problems of refraction are frequent. Myopia as a result of prematurity is a mild complication. The smaller the infant the more significant it is at first, but it all disappears around the age of 1 year. This myopia should be distinguished from that which accompanies the retinal anomalies in the permanent retinopathy that results from hyperoxygenation.

Lesions of scar tissue of the peripheral retina are also frequent and must be screened for systematically in the child born prematurely. They may appear long after birth in an otherwise undamaged child who has had normal funduscopic examination results. There is a retinal pigmentary change that is minimal and benign; it is a sequela of peripheral retinal edema that results in a finely pigmented, atrophic appearance.

Vascular anomalies are common, with the findings of tortuosity, neovascularization, and inequalities in the size of the vessels as conditions that should be followed. *Vitreous changes* are more dangerous; a fibrous preretinal membrane can form folds that may exert dangerous traction on the optic disk, resulting in a deformation.

The pediatrician must therefore be alert to the existence and the significance of these signs and must be able to recognize even the most subtle manifestations of retinopathy of the premature infant, an evolutive disease for which the late complications such as tearing or detachment of the retina must be avoided.

Functional anomalies must also be looked for in the first year. Each eye must be separately screened for *amblyopia* by fixation and following of an object. *Strabismus*, the deviation of the ocular axes, can be noted by position and centering of the corneal reflex.

All ocular deviation after the age of 5 months should be the subject of a specialized examination soon after the initial observation, since early treatment is usually essential for good results. Moreover, the organic anomalies described above are often asymmetric and are manifested by a strabismus; the fundal examination uncovers the etiology of the strabismus as predominantly a unilateral organic anomaly.

In conclusion, the relatively simple ophthalmological examination serves to confirm good visual function, in most cases during the first year. In the rare case where there is doubt as to the existence of an organic lesion or a functional anomaly, an examination under general anesthesia will be indicated, so as to allow an electrophysiological evaluation to be performed, including evoked potentials or an electroretinogram.

AUDITION

There are even stronger differences of opinion about the different mechanisms responsible for the loss of auditory acuity in LBW children: anoxia, jaundice, excessive noise of the incubators. The facts are as follows: on one hand, the frequency of loss of perceptual hearing, moderate to severe, is close to 10% of LBW children, when it is evaluated correctly. The clinical examination is not sufficient [19]. On the other hand, transmission loss is equally frequent in children who have had assisted ventilation because of the inflammatory state of the respiratory tract during the first year. Therefore, a serous otitis media must always be suspected and treated at the first indication of transmission loss.

Mass screening in maternity wards is based on simple clinical methods, demonstrating the cochleomuscular reflex during the first 10 days of life using an acoustic stimulator that utilizes white noise, with pure or modulated sound. The orientation reflex can also be used for screening from the age of 6 months with toys that make sounds. However, this screening is not enough for the population of newborns at risk, particularly newborns weighing <1500 g at birth. It must be understood that up to the age of 5 months, the deaf infant can have vocal behavior identical to the infant who can hear. Therefore, there may not be indications of the problem during the first year.

The postauricular myogenic response (PAM) test described by Fraser *et al.* [20] seems to be a simple and reliable test that can be done during the first year of life. It utilizes the acoustic reflex from the brain stem and seventh and eighth cranial nerves. The perception of sound results in a muscular potential in the posterior auricular muscle, which is detected by a surface electrode [21].

In the case of doubt or a negative result, the child should be sent for a specialized evaluation. Besides careful examination of the eardrum, three other examinations are valuable:

Impedance testing, possible after age 6 months, studies the middle ear, giving a tympanogram; it can detect serous effusions in the middle ear and therefore show that a simple mechanical problem of transmission is responsible for a partial auditory deficit.

Subjective tonal audiometry is possible after age 4 months, examining the two ears simultaneously frequency by frequency, using the method of conditioned reflex orientation. This method allows the confirmation of normal function if the responses are satisfactory, but it does not pick up specific deficits. If the responses have not been satisfactory, it is necessary to investigate further using electrophysiological methods.

Electrophysiological audiometry allows the recording of electric potentials evoked by acoustic stimulation. Use of the electrocochleograph necessitates anesthesia, since the electrode is transtympanic. Brain stem evoked potentials testing necessitates only sedation, so that the child is calm and still. Cortical evoked potentials remain controversial in their interpretation.

The precise results obtained by this group of investigations allows for early use of a mechanical aid, prevents a delay in speech, and prevents problems in adaptation to school. It is therefore essential to screen children at risk systematically and not accept clinical impression of normal hearing, since these specialized investigations can be done very early, during the first year of life.

References

[1] Gesell A. *The mental growth of the preschool child. A psychological outline of normal development from birth to the sixth year including a system of developmental diagnosis.* MacMillan, New York, 1925.

[2] Gesell A. *The first years of life.* Harper & Row, New York, 1940.

[3] Gesell A. *The first five years of life. A guide to the study of the preschool child.* Methuen & Co., London, 1950.

[4] Bayley N. *Bayley Scales of Infant Development manual.* The Psychological Corporation, New York, 1969.

[5] Hunt J. V. and Bayley N. Explorations into patterns of mental development and prediction from the Bayley Scales of Infant Development. In:

Minnesota Symposium on child psychology, J. P. Hill (Ed.), pp. 52–71. University of Minnesota Press, Minneapolis, 1971.

[6] Griffiths R. *The abilities of babies.* University of London Press, London, 1954.

[7] Brunet O. and Lezine I. *Le développement psychologique de la première enfance*, 2nd ed. Presses Universitaires de France, Paris, 1966.

[8] Ramsay M. and Fitzhardinge P. M. A comparative study of two developmental scales: the Bayley and the Griffiths. *Early Hum. Dev.*, *1/2*, 151, 1977.

[9] Uzgiris J. C. and Hunt J. Mc V. *Assessment in infancy; ordinal scales of psychological development.* University of Illinois Press, Chicago, 1975.

[10] McCall R. B. Predicting developmental outcome, résumé and redirection. In: *New approaches to developmental screening of infants*, T. B. Brazelton and B. M. Lester (Eds.), pp. 13–26. Elsevier, New York, 1983.

[11] Sower T. G. R. *A primer of infant development.* Freeman & Co, San Francisco, 1977.

[12] Parmelee A. H. and Schulte F. J. Developmental testing of preterm and small for date infants. *Pediatrics*, *45*, 21, 1970.

[13] Hunt J. V. Longitudinal research: a method for studying the intellectual development of high-risk preterm infants. In: *Infants born at risk: behavior and development*, T. M. Field, A. M. Sostek, S. Goldberg and H. H. Shuman (Eds.), pp. 443–460. Spectrum Publications, London, 1979.

[14] Fitzhardinge P. M. Current outcome of NICU population. In: *Neonatal neurological assessment and outcome: report of the seventy-seventh Ross Conference on pediatric research*, A. W. Brann and J. J. Volpe (Eds). Ross Laboratories, Columbus, 1980.

[15] Hunt J. V., Tooley W. H. and Harvin D. Learning disabilities in children with birth weights ≤1500 grams. *Semin. Perinatol.*, *6*, 280–287, 1982.

[16] Drillien C. M., Thomson A. J. M. and Burgoyne K. Low birth weight children at early school-age: a longitudinal study. *Dev. Med. Child Neurol.*, *22*, 26, 1980.

[17] Silverman W. A. *Retrolental fibroplasia, a modern paradox. Monographs in Neonatology.* Grune & Stratton, New York, 1980.

[18] Silverman W. A. Retinopathy of prematurity: oxygen dogma challenged. *Arch. Dis. Child.*, *57*, 731–733, 1982.

[19] Abramovitch S. J., Gregory S., Slemick M. and Steward A. Hearing loss in very low birth weight infants treated with neonatal intensive care. *Arch. Dis. Child.*, *54*, 421–426, 1979.

[20] Fraser J. C., Conway M. J., Keene M. H. and Hazell J. W. P. The post-auricular myogenic response: a new instrument which simplifies its detection by machine scoring. *J. Laryngol. Otol.*, *92*, 293–303, 1978.

[21] Hope P. L., Hazell J. W. P. and Stewart A. L. Sensorineural hearing loss in the very low birth weight survivor. In: *Proceedings of the Scientific Meetings of the Bristol Association of Audiological Physicians.* I. G. Taylor (Ed.), Manchester, 1981, pp. 23–37. Publ. Dept. of Audiology and Education, University of Manchester, 1982.

8

CONCLUSIONS

Two questions come to mind at the end of this monograph.

After having followed infants at risk from before birth to 1 year and collected data up to primary school, the first question is: what about adulthood? Jane McFarlane, a pioneer of the Berkeley study, once ended a dinner conversation with this comment: "What is interesting with human beings is how unpredictable they are." As she worked in Berkeley and stayed on after retirement, and remained in touch with a number of people included in the study, she was able to maintain contact into the second and sometimes third generations. She could remember that the boy with the highest IQ she had ever met became a policeman in Arizona, and that many moderately handicapped children did very well later on in life. There does not seem to be much point, therefore, in continuing routine follow-up into adolescence.

After having classified infants at risk into three groups, the second question is: is it worthwhile to create such separations in a continuum, and what does the pediatrician hope to achieve in doing so? Let us look at the three groups down the road:

1. A *severely damaged* child will remain so throughout his life. Grenier's answer to the question of brain plasticity in severe handicaps is, "Fifteen years after creating an institution for handicapped children, I had to create another one for handicapped adults."

2. A fetus or a newborn at risk has to prove very early in life that risk does not mean abnormality. The newborn infant is urged to demonstrate that he is normal, absolutely normal. He can do this in the first weeks of life and confirm it at 2 years. In this way, and only in this way, can a competent newborn and his competent pediatrician calm parents' anxieties.

3. There are a lot of infants in between the normal and severely handicapped categories; they are the ones with *minimal brain dysfunction*. For most of them Rapin predicts a decent adulthood. This prediction will help both the child and his parents to weather the storm:*

> Since school is, for the majority of persons, the most severe test of their cognitive abilities, many brain-damaged and mildly retarded persons will be less conspicuous as adults than as children. Those who have acquired adequate social skills, learned a trade, and found a niche in the marketplace, that does not penalize them too severely for their deficits, and those who do not have severe emotional problems, and do not engage in antisocial behavior are likely to disappear into the population.

Therefore, we feel that the pediatrician who is able to provide the obstetrician and intensive care workers with short-term data classified into three groups—normal, acceptable, and severely damaged—will help them evaluate their progress in perinatology.

*Rapin I. *Children with brain dysfunction*. Raven Press, New York, 1982, p. 211.

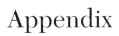

Appendix

1

NEUROLOGIC   EVALUATION – AMIEL-TISON

RECORD FORM FOR MONTHLY EXAMINATION WITHIN THE FIRST YEAR

NAME   SEX

DATE OF BIRTH

GESTATIONAL AGE   [   ]   WEEKS

CORRECTION FACTOR 40–G.A. = [   ]   WEEKS

DATE	PRESENT AGE	CORRECTED AGE	EXAMINATION NUMBER	TESTED BY

HEAD CIRCUMFERENCE (see growth curves)

	1	2	3	4	5	6	7	8	9	10	11	12
cm												
+2 SD												
-2 SD												

ANTERIOR FONTANELLE

Normal

Tense

Depressed

SUTURES

Normal

Separated

Overlapping

USUAL PATTERN FOR WAKEFULNESS AND SLEEP

Normal

Agitated, too much crying

Lethargic, no crying

ESTIMATION OF ALERTNESS DURING THE TEST

Satisfactory

Constantly agitated

Lethargic

CRY

Normal

High-pitched

Weak

Monotonous

Other

| | 1 | 2 | 3 | 4 | 5 | 6 | 7 | 8 | 9 | 10 | 11 | 12 |

SUCKING BEHAVIOUR

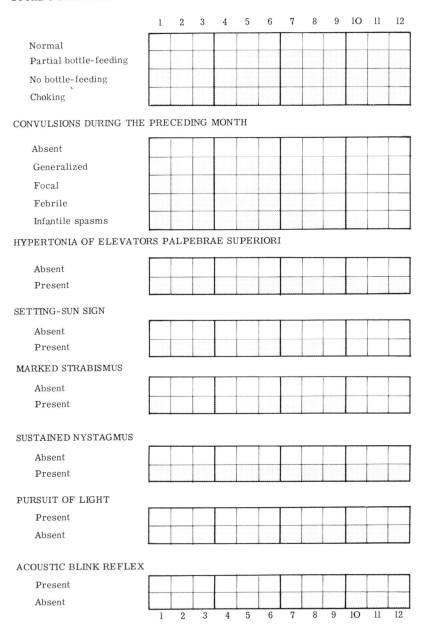

	1	2	3	4	5	6	7	8	9	10	11	12
Normal												
Partial bottle-feeding												
No bottle-feeding												
Choking												

CONVULSIONS DURING THE PRECEDING MONTH

| Absent |
| Generalized |
| Focal |
| Febrile |
| Infantile spasms |

HYPERTONIA OF ELEVATORS PALPEBRAE SUPERIORI

| Absent |
| Present |

SETTING-SUN SIGN

| Absent |
| Present |

MARKED STRABISMUS

| Absent |
| Present |

SUSTAINED NYSTAGMUS

| Absent |
| Present |

PURSUIT OF LIGHT

| Present |
| Absent |

ACOUSTIC BLINK REFLEX

| Present |
| Absent |

| | 1 | 2 | 3 | 4 | 5 | 6 | 7 | 8 | 9 | 10 | 11 | 12 |

ASYMMETRIC TONIC NECK REFLEX (POSTURAL)

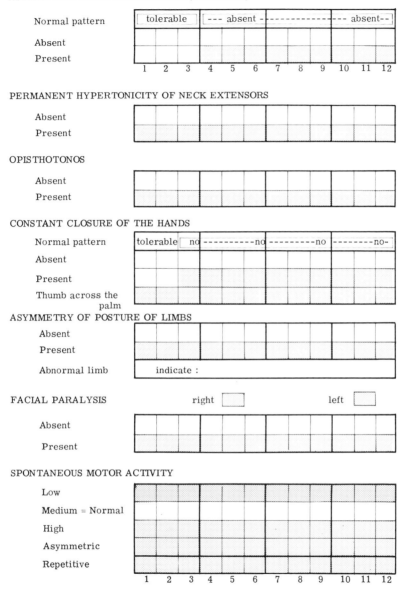

Normal pattern   tolerable   --- absent ------------- absent--

Absent

Present

    1   2   3   4   5   6   7   8   9   10   11   12

PERMANENT HYPERTONICITY OF NECK EXTENSORS

Absent

Present

OPISTHOTONOS

Absent

Present

CONSTANT CLOSURE OF THE HANDS

Normal pattern   tolerable   no ----------no ---------no --------no-

Absent

Present

Thumb across the palm

ASYMMETRY OF POSTURE OF LIMBS

Absent

Present

Abnormal limb   indicate :

FACIAL PARALYSIS   right   left

Absent

Present

SPONTANEOUS MOTOR ACTIVITY

Low

Medium = Normal

High

Asymmetric

Repetitive

    1   2   3   4   5   6   7   8   9   10   11   12

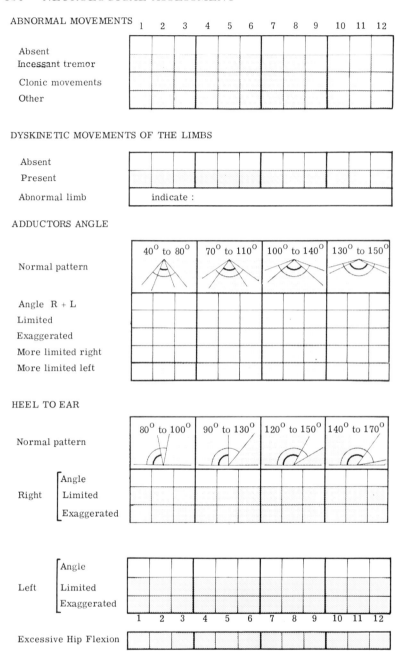

ABNORMAL MOVEMENTS

	1	2	3	4	5	6	7	8	9	10	11	12
Absent												
Incessant tremor												
Clonic movements												
Other												

DYSKINETIC MOVEMENTS OF THE LIMBS

Absent	
Present	
Abnormal limb	indicate :

ADDUCTORS ANGLE

	40° to 80°	70° to 110°	100° to 140°	130° to 150°
Normal pattern				
Angle R + L				
Limited				
Exaggerated				
More limited right				
More limited left				

HEEL TO EAR

	80° to 100°	90° to 130°	120° to 150°	140° to 170°
Normal pattern				
Right [Angle				
Limited				
Exaggerated]				

Left [Angle	
Limited	
Exaggerated]	

	1	2	3	4	5	6	7	8	9	10	11	12

Excessive Hip Flexion

POPLITEAL ANGLE

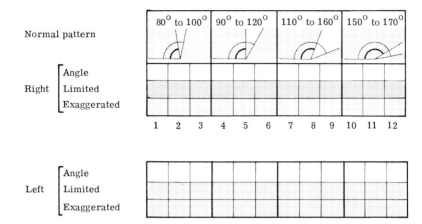

Normal pattern

Right: Angle / Limited / Exaggerated

Left: Angle / Limited / Exaggerated

DORSIFLEXION ANGLE OF THE FOOT

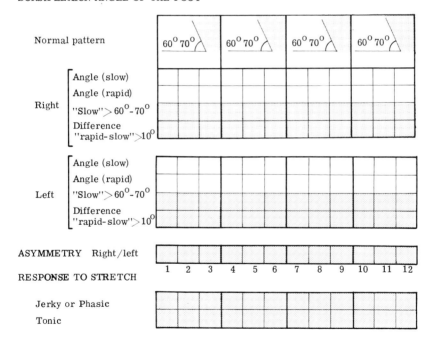

Normal pattern

Right: Angle (slow) / Angle (rapid) / "Slow" > 60°-70° / Difference "rapid-slow" > 10°

Left: Angle (slow) / Angle (rapid) / "Slow" > 60°-70° / Difference "rapid-slow" > 10°

ASYMMETRY   Right/left

RESPONSE TO STRETCH

Jerky or Phasic

Tonic

SCARF SIGN

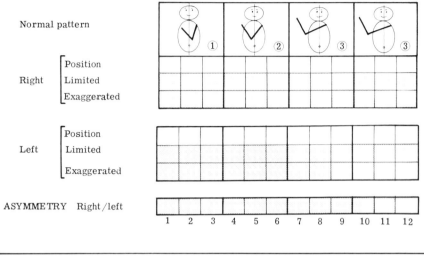

Normal pattern

Right — Position / Limited / Exaggerated

Left — Position / Limited / Exaggerated

ASYMMETRY   Right/left

1   2   3   4   5   6   7   8   9   10   11   12

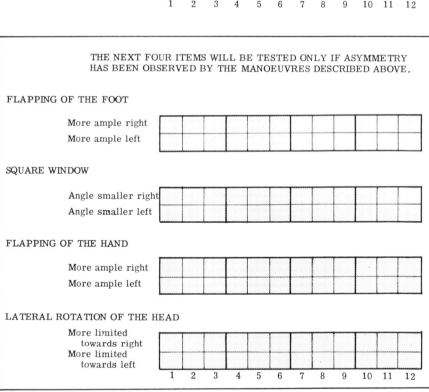

THE NEXT FOUR ITEMS WILL BE TESTED ONLY IF ASYMMETRY
HAS BEEN OBSERVED BY THE MANOEUVRES DESCRIBED ABOVE.

FLAPPING OF THE FOOT

More ample right
More ample left

SQUARE WINDOW

Angle smaller right
Angle smaller left

FLAPPING OF THE HAND

More ample right
More ample left

LATERAL ROTATION OF THE HEAD

More limited
towards right
More limited
towards left

1   2   3   4   5   6   7   8   9   10   11   12

REPEATED VENTRAL FLEXION OF THE HEAD

Identical

More stiffness

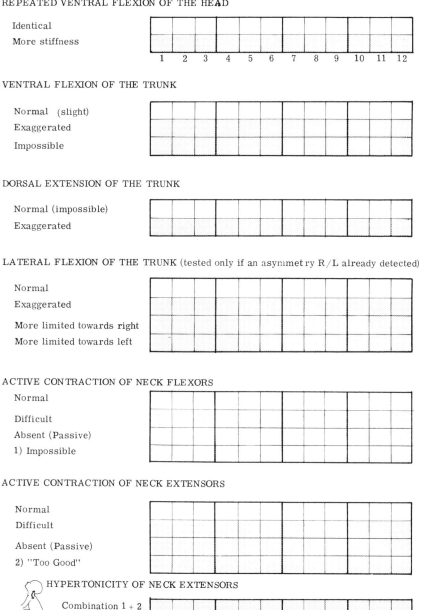

1   2   3   4   5   6   7   8   9   10   11   12

VENTRAL FLEXION OF THE TRUNK

Normal (slight)

Exaggerated

Impossible

DORSAL EXTENSION OF THE TRUNK

Normal (impossible)

Exaggerated

LATERAL FLEXION OF THE TRUNK (tested only if an asymmetry R/L already detected)

Normal

Exaggerated

More limited towards right

More limited towards left

ACTIVE CONTRACTION OF NECK FLEXORS

Normal

Difficult

Absent (Passive)

1) Impossible

ACTIVE CONTRACTION OF NECK EXTENSORS

Normal

Difficult

Absent (Passive)

2) "Too Good"

HYPERTONICITY OF NECK EXTENSORS

Combination 1 + 2

1   2   3   4   5   6   7   8   9   10   11   12

HEAD CONTROL

Normal Pattern	absent	inconstant	--------- present ----------
Present			
Absent			

PULLS TO SITTING POSITION

	1	2	3	4	5	6	7	8	9	10	11	12
Normal pattern	absent				inconstant			present				
Present												
Absent												

SITS ALONE MOMENTARILY

Normal pattern	absent		inconstant		present	
Present						
Collapses forward						
Falls backward						

SITS ALONE 30 SECONDS OR MORE

Normal pattern	absent		inconstant		present	
Present						
Absent						

STRAIGHTENING WITH LOWER LIMBS AND TRUNK   (supporting reaction)

Normal pattern	Present	inconstant	-absent	---	Possible not sustained	Present
Present						
Absent						
Scissoring						
Trunk arching						
	1 2	3 4	5 6	7	8 9	10 11 12

AUTOMATIC WALKING

Normal pattern

| present | inconstant | ------- absent ---------- |

Present
Absent

1   2   3   4   5   6   7   8   9   10   11   12

PALMAR GRASP

Normal pattern

| present | inconstant | ---------- absent ----------- |

Present
Absent
Asymmetry R/L

RESPONSE TO TRACTION

Normal pattern

| present | inconstant | ---------- absent ----------- |

Present
Absent
Asymmetry R/L

MORO REFLEX

Normal pattern

| present | inconstant | ---------- absent -------- |

Present
Absent
Asymmetry R/L
Clonic movements
+ low threshold

ABNORMAL LIMB IN THE LAST 4 MANOEUVRES

[   ] Right   [   ] Left

ASYMMETRIC TONIC NECK REFLEX (evoked)

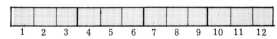

1   2   3   4   5   6   7   8   9   10   11   12

BICEPS REFLEX

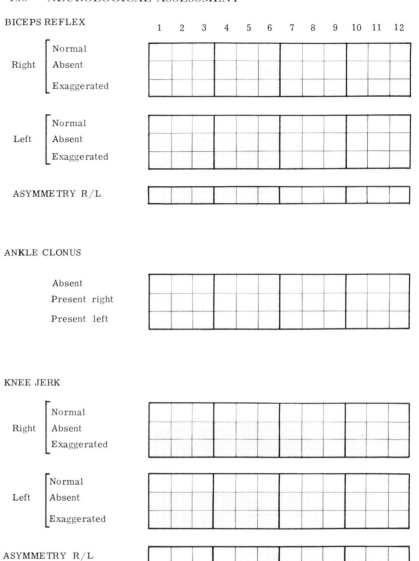

Right
- Normal
- Absent
- Exaggerated

Left
- Normal
- Absent
- Exaggerated

ASYMMETRY R/L

ANKLE CLONUS

- Absent
- Present right
- Present left

KNEE JERK

Right
- Normal
- Absent
- Exaggerated

Left
- Normal
- Absent
- Exaggerated

ASYMMETRY R/L

LATERAL PROPPING REACTION

Normal pattern	-- absent ---	-- absent ---	inconst- ant	--- -- present -
Present				
Absent				
Asymmetry R/L				

PARACHUTE

	1	2	3	4	5	6	7	8	9	10	11	12
Normal pattern	-- absent ---			-- absent ---		---		inconst- ant		-- present -		
Present												
Absent												
Asymmetry R/L												

Abnormal limb in the last 2 manoeuvres   ☐ right   ☐ left

CLINICAL IMPRESSION DURING THE FIRST YEAR

	1 - 3	4 - 6	7 - 9	10-12
MICROCEPHALUS intra-uterine post-natal				
HYDROCEPHALUS intra-uterine post-natal				
HYPEREXCITABILITY (irritable, restless sleep pattern, abnormal movements, low threshold for primary reflexes, upper eye-lid hypertonia, persistent fisting).				
LETHARGY (sleepy and difficult to waken, reduced spontaneous movements, infrequent crying, poor or absent primary reflexes).				
ABNORMALITIES OF PASSIVE TONE 1) Global hypotonia ("floppy baby", trunk and limbs).				
2) Upper body hypotonia (weak neck flexion, exaggerated scarf sign, poor response to traction).				
3) Flexion hypertonia of lower limbs (persistence of neonatal angles, adductor, heel to ear, popliteal).				
4) Flexion hypertonia of upper limbs (persistent fisting and limited scarf sign).				
5) Imbalance in passive tone of trunk (reduced ventral flexion + increased dorsal extention).				
6) Asymmetric tone (hemisyndrom)				

Months

	1 - 3	4 - 6	7 - 9	10-12
ABNORMALITIES OF ACTIVE TONE				
1) Hyperactivity of neck extensors (head unable to drop forward).				
2) Hyperactivity of neck and trunk extensors (arching)				
3) Poor active tone, "floppy baby" (no head control, no sitting position, no standing position - according to normal pattern).				

PERIPHERAL NERVE PALSY
   face
   limbs				

DELAYED APPEARANCE OF POSTURAL REACTIONS (lateral propping and parachute).				
IMPAIRED HEARING				
STRABISMUS				
OTHER OCULAR ABNORMALITIES				
DEVELOPMENTAL DELAY (test or subtest).				

SEIZURES
   febrile
   nonfebrile				

EEG ABNORMALITY				

Months

Name

Date of Birth

G.A.

Birth-weight

SUMMARY AT THE END
OF THE FIRST YEAR

NO ABNORMALITY

PATTERNS OF TRANSIENT ABNORMALITIES

1) Hyperexcitability
   Hypertonia of neck extensors ☐

2) Hypotonia. Lethargy
   Primary reflexes poor or absent ☐

3) Mimmicking spastic diplegia ☐
   (no relaxation in lower limbs,
   poor active tone, persisting primary
   reflexes, phasic contraction to stretch,
   exaggerated deep tendon reflexes).

4) Mimmicking spastic hemiplegia ☐
   (no relaxation on one side, asymmetric
   movements, exaggerated deep tendon
   reflexes).

5) Mimmicking spastic quadriplegia ☐

6) Developmental delay ☐
   (global or subtest abnormality).

7) Miscellaneous ☐

PATTERNS OF PERSISTENT ABNORMALITIES

1) Cerebral palsy   spastic diplegia
                     spastic hemiplegia   ☐
                     quadriplegia
                     choreoathetosis

2) Microcephalus ☐

3) Hydrocephalus ☐

4) Mental retardation ☐

5) Convulsions   febrile
                  non febrile   ☐

6) Sensory problems   auditory
                       visual   ☐

7) Miscellaneous ☐

ETIOLOGY

Genetic   certain ☐   Perinatal   pre-natal ☐   Miscellaneous ☐
           probable ☐   intra-partum ☐
                                       post-natal ☐   Unknown ☐

INDEX

195